Eugene Perkowski 01/10/02

SAVE YOUR ACHING BACK

A Patient's Guide

by

Stewart G. Eidelson, M.D.
Gregory Gilreath, P.A.-C.
Michael Whitehurst, Ed.D.

SYA Press, Inc.

Published by:
SYA Press, Inc., 1355 West Palmetto Park Road, Suite 115,
Boca Raton, Florida, 33486.

DISCLAIMER:
Every effort has been made by the authors to provide the most accurate information possible. However, this book is not all-inclusive. This book is not intended to replace the relationship between the reader and their physician or medical professional. Therefore, the reader assumes all responsibility and risks in the use of the information contained herein. Neither the authors, collaborators, SYA Press, Inc., the Palm Beach Orthopaedic & Spinal Research Foundation, nor the South Florida Orthopaedic Group shall be held responsible for errors, omissions in information herein, or liable for damages resulting in whole or in part from this material.

Library of Congress Cataloging-in-Publication Data

Eidelson, M.D., Stewart G., 1950-
Save your aching back, a patient's guide
Stewart G. Eidelson, M.D.-1st ed.
Includes biographical references and index.
ISBN 0-9669252-0-3

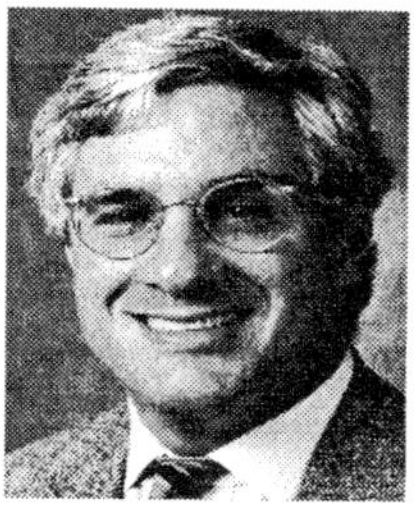

STEWART G. EIDELSON, M.D.

Dr. Eidelson is a 1972 graduate of Drew University in Madison, New Jersey with a degree in Zoology. He graduated from Thomas Jefferson Medical College in Philadelphia, Pennsylvania in 1976, and served his internship at Metropolitan Hospital in New York. His orthopaedic surgery residences were completed at the Geisinger Medical Center in Danville, Pennsylvania, and the Alfred I. duPont Institute in Wilmington, Delaware.

He received advanced Fellowship Training in Spinal Surgery at the Cleveland Spine Center under the direction of Dr. Arthur Steffee, and was on the teaching faculty of the Shriners Hospital for Crippled Children in Lexington, Kentucky for seven years.

Dr. Eidelson is a member of the North American Spine Society, the Palm Beach County Medical Society, the Florida Orthopaedic Society, and the Palm Beach County Orthopaedic Society. Dr. Eidelson is Board Certified by the American Board of Orthopaedic Surgery and is a Fellow of the American Academy of Orthopaedic Surgeons.

continued...

Stewart G. Eidelson, M.D. continued...

With his keen interest in outcome studies relating to spinal surgical procedures in the elderly, Dr. Eidelson was instrumental in founding the Palm Beach Orthopaedic and Spinal Research Foundation located in Boca Raton, Florida. In conjunction with the Foundation's research, many of Dr. Eidelson's papers have been accepted and presented worldwide.

Additionally, Dr. Eidelson engages in ongoing public forums in South Florida. These informative forums allow dynamic interaction with patients and their family members, and other interested people in the community. These experiences, as well as a large spinal care nonsurgical and surgical practice, allow him to bring key issues regarding back disorders to the forefront.

♦ ♦ ♦ ♦ ♦

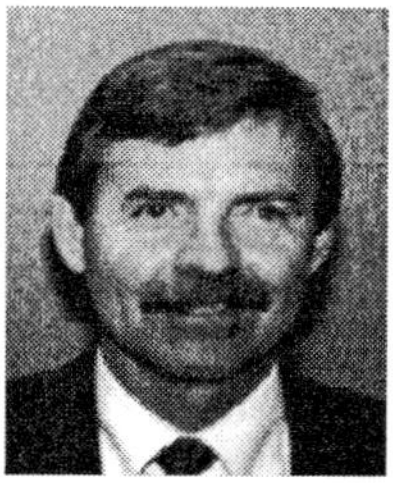

GREGORY GILREATH, P.A.-C.

Mr. Gilreath is Dr. Eidelson's Physician's Assistant and serves as the Palm Beach Orthopaedic and Spinal Research Foundation's Administrator. Mr. Gilreath has 36 years of medical experience, 26 of which has been dedicated to orthopaedic spinal surgery.

As a former Cincinnati native and graduate from the University of Cincinnati, Mr. Gilreath received degrees in Zoology and Psychology, and training in surgical technology. He received neurologic orthopaedic training at the Mayfield Neurological Institute in Cincinnati, Ohio.

Additionally, Mr. Gilreath trained under Dr. Arthur Steffee and Dr. John Collis, both spine specialists in Cleveland, Ohio. He also received specialized instruction under Dr. Gabriel Ma and Dr. Ralph Cloward (one of the 'founding Fathers' of spinal surgery) in Honolulu, Hawaii, and Dr. Charles Edwards from Johns Hopkins University in Baltimore, Maryland.

♦ ♦ ♦ ♦ ♦

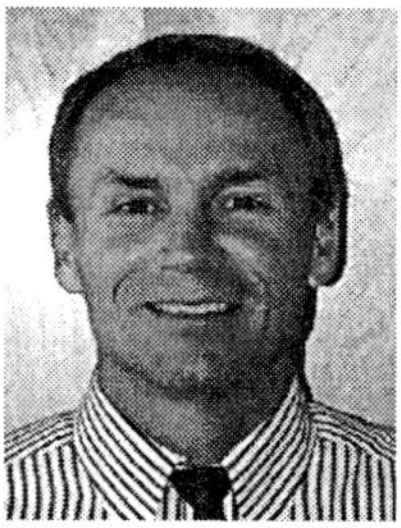

MICHAEL WHITEHURST, Ed.D.

Dr. Whitehurst is a Professor and Associate Dean at Florida Atlantic University's College of Education. In addition, Dr. Whitehurst assisted with the development of the University's new physical therapy program in the Health Sciences Department.

In 1975, he received a B.S. degree in Exercise Science/ Biology from the University of Arizona. While attending the University of Georgia, in 1978 he received his M.Ed. and his Ed.D. in 1981, both in Exercise Science.

His research work is comprehensive, including several grant proposals, as well as more than 100 publications and presentations. His contributions to the Palm Beach Orthopaedic and Spinal Research Foundation continue to be extensive.

♦ ♦ ♦ ♦ ♦

TABLE OF CONTENTS

	.... Introduction	i - iv
Chapter 1....	You Are Not Alone!	Page 1
Chapter 2....	A Short Lesson in Spinal Anatomy	Page 7
Chapter 3....	Consulting A Specialist and The Diagnosis	Page 27
Chapter 4....	Diagnostic Tests	Page 36
Chapter 5....	Common Spinal Disorders	Page 45
Chapter 6....	Managing The Pain	Page 87
Chapter 7....	Physical Therapy	Page 92
Chapter 8....	Alternative Therapies	Page 108
Chapter 9....	If All Else Fails ... Spinal Surgery	Page 111
	.... Authors' Last Words	Page 136
Chapter 10...	Glossary of Terms	Page 137
	.... Index	Page 151

ILLUSTRATIONS

2.1	Anterior View, Spinal Column	Page 11
2.2	Posterior View, Spinal Column	Page 13
2.3	Lateral View, Spinal Column	Page 14
2.3B	Section of Lateral Spine	Page 15
2.4	Normal Vertebral Disc	Page 17
2.5	Interior, Spinal Cord	Page 19
2.6	Lateral View, Spinal Cord	Page 20
2.7	Posterior View, Spinal Cord	Page 21
2.8	Dermatomes	Page 22
2.9	Posterior View, Spine & Muscles	Page 25
3.1	Pain Diagram	Page 30
5.1	Sciatic Nerve	Page 52
5.2	Fracture	Page 56
5.3	Spondylolisthesis	Page 60
5.4	Scoliosis	Page 64

Illustrations Continued...

Illustrations Continued ...

5.5	Kyphosis	Page 65
5.6	Lordosis	Page 66
5.7	Herniated Disc	Page 69
5.8	Bulging Disc	Page 70
5.9	Bone Spurs or Bony Overgrowths	Page 73
5.10	Osteoarthritis	Page 75
5.11	Spinal Stenosis	Page 78
5.12	Degenerative Disc Disease	Page 81
5.13	Osteoporosis	Page 85
7.1	Proper Posture	Page 102
9.1	Laminotomy	Page 125
9.2	Laminectomy	Page 126
9.3	Spinal Instrumentation and Fusion	Page 130
9.4	The 'CAGE'	Page 131

To Elizabeth, David, and Sarah with love.

ACKNOWLEDGMENTS

This book could not have been written without the collaborative efforts of Gregory Gilreath, P.A.-C. and Dr. Michael Whitehurst. Without their experience, support, and limitless hours of editing, this book would still be just an idea.

As we approached the end of this project, Dr. George J. Kolettis and Dr. Richard Lieberman assisted by offering their editorial support. We are grateful for their advice as we prepared for publication.

Gratitude is also extended to Dana Davis, M.P.T., Shari Herschenhorn, R.P.T., and Alexandra Kalnitsky, M.A. for their physical therapy expertise. Despite significant patient responsibilities, they were each able to adjust their schedules to help 'fine tune' Chapter 7. Ms. Herschenhorn provided a wealth of information pertaining to the patient's initial evaluation and its importance. Thanks to Ms. Davis, we were able to accurately describe the difference between modalities and other forms of treatment. The question "How do you prepare a treatment plan?" was answered in part by Ms. Kalnitsky. In addition, she was able to demonstrate the benefits of specific exercises and rehab programs.

Dr. Richard Tiegen, D.M.D., A.P., the Director of the Wellness Center for the South Florida Orthopaedic Group, is responsible for contributing to the section on acupuncture and its importance as an alternative therapy.

Acknowledgments continued ...

Acknowledgments continued ...

Furthermore, without the efforts of Susan Spinasanta, a professional writer, this book would still be a jumble of ideas. She organized our thoughts into meaningful sentences, gracefully forced us to sit down to pour over drafts, and pulled the loose ends together.

We would also like to say 'thank you' to our three area hospitals: Bethesda Memorial Hospital in Boynton Beach, Boca Raton Community Hospital in Boca Raton, and Delray Community Hospital in Delray Beach. We greatly appreciate the opportunity to be affiliated with these fine hospitals.

INTRODUCTION

About a year ago, I was sitting in a local bookstore waiting for my children. For over an hour I watched as different people came to stand around reading medical books and then moved on to leave space for other interested readers. As a physician, I was naturally curious to know what they were reading. So I wandered in their direction to peek over a shoulder or two. I could hardly believe it. Each person was reading about some aspect of back care!

Without revealing my identity, I casually asked a few individuals if they were finding answers to their questions. In the end, I determined these people were looking for simple answers to their questions ... the same types of questions my patients have been asking for 15 years!

Although I have considered writing this book for years, the time spent at the bookstore helped me to develop its purpose: *a book specifically written in 'lay-person language' designed to meet the needs of the average person with back trouble.*

I can't thank my children enough for dragging me to the bookstore that afternoon!

♦ ♦ ♦ ♦ ♦

It may be said, that the pathway to finding relief from a back problem may present many twists and turns. There are chiropractors, physical therapists, primary care doctors, and even internists treating back pain. Then there are neurosurgeons, orthopaedic surgeons, and rheumatologists. Finding the right physician to treat a back disorder is simply not the same as treating chest pain.

Consider this ... a cardiologist would treat someone with an abnormal EKG. A urologist would treat a bladder disorder. But what about a patient with burning pain radiating from the buttock down into the thigh? Who does this patient consult?

The reader should view this book as his or her navigational tool through uncertain waters. One of the objectives of this book is to try to map out an easy to follow guide for patients. *Save Your Aching Back, A Patient's Guide* has been written to answer typical questions and to enhance the reader's general level of understanding. We are hopeful this knowledge may lead to a more productive visit with the doctor or therapist.

This book is composed of 10 concisely written chapters that follow a logical course beginning with basic spinal anatomy. Illustrations are provided throughout the book to enhance the reader's understanding of the text. Glancing through the pages of this book, the reader will find that medical terminology has been translated into a language easy to understand.

Additionally, many of the medical terms have been phonetically spelled to benefit pronunciation. For quick reference, a **Glossary** is provided toward the end of the book.

The reader will learn what to expect during an office consultation and the role of diagnostic testing. Emphasis has been placed on the importance of a correct diagnosis followed by a discussion relating to **Common Spinal Disorders**. After a diagnosis has been made, the next step is treatment. Some treatment plans may include pain management. Physical therapy may be an important component to help restore the patient's functional ability, as well as alternative therapies such as acupuncture and biofeedback.

Surgery may be considered a possible option *only* after conservative treatment options have *absolutely* failed. Some patients may find it comforting to know that out of approximately 100 patients, fewer than 5% may require surgery. Additionally, in many cases, surgery is not done on an emergency basis. Therefore, the patient may have time to discuss the procedure with his or her spinal surgeon and other physicians.

Many of the points covered in this book address the questions and concerns raised by patients who have attended any of our public symposiums. These monthly symposiums enable us to inform the public about the findings from research conducted by the Palm Beach Orthopaedic and Spinal Research Foundation.

The Foundation, dedicated to the advancement of spinal research, was formed five years ago. Through its support of our public forums, we have been able to report technological improvements made in orthopaedic medicine, specifically those relating to spinal disorders.

Also, the Palm Beach Orthopaedic and Spinal Research Foundation is an organization committed to the study of functional outcomes. An *outcome* refers to the patient's functional ability following treatment for a spinal disorder. One of the Foundation's goals is to sponsor research addressing the extent to which patients benefit functionally following non-surgical or surgical intervention. For example, a particular research project was aimed at answering questions such as "Does this procedure work?" ... "Are we in fact in an objective way providing the best care and treatment?" ... "Is this being accurately assessed?". To this end, the Foundation has relied on Dr. Michael Whitehurst, a Professor and Associate Dean in Florida Atlantic University's College of Education, to design and implement studies of functional outcomes.

My staff and I continue to routinely administer our tests to back patients. These tests and outcomes have been published and presented worldwide. All of this work substantiates the Foundation's mission to discover, analyze, prove, and share the results for the global advancement of spinal research.

Stewart G. Eidelson, M.D.

♦ ♦ ♦ ♦ ♦

1-58-DG
BROSS-

BROSS - 158

MARYSIA + JUREK

6

001 48222 240189

BROSS GABRIELT SYLVIA

158 SEVILLE G.

496-5100

2

Publix®

G (BOSS)

ALAW

Chapter 1

You Are Not Alone!

Joe and Lillian, like many people their age, vacation in Florida during the cold northern winters. During the drive south, Joe daydreams about golf and improving his handicap. No sooner have they arrived, than the car is unpacked and Joe is on the golf course with his buddies.

Later that evening, Joe's lower back begins to ache. He brushes the pain off as simply the price paid for a near perfect game of golf. However, several days later while in the doctor's office, Joe complains that he can't understand why his back *still* aches.

♦ ♦ ♦ ♦ ♦

Does Joe's problem sound familiar? Actually, what happened to Joe is quite common. Although his problem was not serious, his absence from playing golf may be to blame. He hadn't been using the back muscles necessary to execute each perfect swing for a few months. Joe's unconditioned muscles were simply not prepared to repeat the golf swing over and over as is required during 18 holes.

Joe's case is just one example why back pain is prevalent in America. At any given time, upward of 60% of the adult population in the United States may be affected by a back disorder. So if you find yourself among the 60%, you certainly are not alone.

As human beings, we have many things in common that may play important roles in the health of our spinal columns. Heredity is one aspect. Scoliosis (sko-lee-oh-sis) is an example of a spinal disorder that may run in families. This disease causes the spine to curve from side to side. If scoliosis is diagnosed early, steps can be taken that may help to control the disease. Individually, our family trees may reveal many clues to our future health. This is one reason why doctors ask about family history.

Even if we don't inherit a tendency toward a particular disease, we all age. Unfortunately, there is no magic pill or treatment that stops this natural process. Here, too, heredity can play a part in an individual's longevity. If your parents and grandparents lived long lives and you inherited those good genes, you may live longer. However, living longer does not guarantee any particular quality of life because the effects from fighting gravity may be more pronounced in some people.

Along with the growing number of older people in America, attitudes about aging are changing. People of all ages are looking for ways to prolong life, stay healthy, and remain active. It wasn't too long ago that retired people were expected to sit on the porch and rock away the years, basically living sedentary lives.

Now we find our grandparents have left the porch, exchanging their rocking chairs for exercise equipment and gym shoes. Older people are participating in the Olympics, marathon races, and competitive sports such as tennis.

Longevity has also increased due to improvement in public health measures such as community sanitation and immunization programs. Medicine has helped to add new drugs to control health problems that at one time may have meant certain death. The discovery of penicillin was the forerunner to the development of antibiotics, which are used today to treat infections that may occur in the spine.

The quality of life has been and continues to be improved for many people with skeletal disorders. In orthopaedics, the wear and tear on older knees and hips may be remedied by replacement. In some cases, age is no longer a barrier to simple or complex surgical procedures necessary to correct a spinal disorder. For example, older patients may receive surgical treatment to relieve the effects of spinal stenosis or degenerative disc disease, as well as other disorders that affect the spine.

Today we are learning that some diseases may result from exposure to environmental hazards. The spine is not exempt because it depends on circulation for oxygen, nourishment, and other elements. The ability to keep our body systems working effectively may be related to the air we breathe and our food sources.

Unfortunately, many environmental hazards, such as air pollution, often cannot be avoided. Some hazards are unknown at the time of exposure. Any form or type of chemical pollutant may negatively affect any body part (i.e. eyes) or system (i.e. respiratory).

The effect of a toxin depends on the type of toxic agent that enters the body, as well as how it is metabolized and eliminated. The liver and kidneys act as the body's filtration systems. An accumulation of toxic agents may eventually prevent these organs from functioning properly. It is now known that certain chemical toxins can alter the genetic code, which could affect future generations.

Speaking of toxins, did you know that one cigarette contains hundreds of chemicals? One of these chemicals, nicotine, is not only addictive, but is considered toxic. Smoking is detrimental to the spine because it can decrease the oxygen supply and upset the nutritional composition of blood, which bones depend on for nourishment. Nicotine can cause blood vessels to constrict, which slows circulation. This is one reason why people who smoke cigarettes, cigars, or a pipe may heal at a slower rate than nonsmokers do.

Children may mimic the behavior of adults they favor. These behaviors may include, unfortunately, smoking cigarettes. During a youngster's formative years, smoking could be a factor contributing to stunting the child's growth. At any age, bones need the nourishment supplied by proper circulation. Additionally, smoking, as well as other factors, could lead to osteoporosis (os-tea-oh-pour-oh-sis), a disease that causes bones to lose strength. People who *choose* to smoke may be placed at a higher risk for spine-related problems.

Overeating is a habit that may lead to obesity. Not only does obesity force the cardiovascular system to work harder, but too much weight may create unnecessary stress to the spine.

Unfortunately, in some cases, obesity may lead to a sedentary lifestyle lacking regular exercise. The spine and its components were designed for activity. If the muscles supporting the spinal column are not used and/or conditioned, they may atrophy.

The spine needs and depends on strong muscles to support the body and execute movement. This is why physical therapy may be incorporated into a treatment plan. Physical therapy helps to condition and strengthen muscles in order to restore functional ability, which may help the patient to return to golf, swimming, tennis, or other activities.

We may not have a fountain of youth to keep us from feeling the effects from growing older, but we do have the ability to learn how to keep our bodies working at maximum capacity.

The following chapter discusses the anatomy of the spine. Learning about the basic components may help you to appreciate why the choices you make are important in an effort to avoid spinal disease or dysfunction.

♦ ♦ ♦ ♦ ♦

Chapter 2

A Short Lesson in Spinal Anatomy

The human skeleton is composed of 206 bones, 33 of which are located in the spine. Bones are long, flat, short or irregularly shaped, and some are thicker than others. Bones are flexible during youth, eventually becoming rigid at maturity. If a bone is broken, *collagen* (coll-ah-gin), which is manufactured by the body, mends the fracture. The new bone is then hardened through a process termed *calcification* (kals-eye-fi-cay-shun).

Bone is a living organ comparable to the heart or kidneys. It contains blood vessels and is nourished through circulation. If any bone or organ system is ignored or misused, it can decay and cause problems.

Within bone are two compartments. The outer layer is termed *cortical* (core-tea-cul) bone and the inner is *cancellous* (cancel-luss) bone. Microscopically, cortical bone looks like concentric rings. Cancellous bone resembles latticework and is spongy. A system of blood vessels supplies the bones with needed nutrition.

Bones serve as storehouses for minerals and fats. Approximately a quarter of a bone's weight is fluid. Minerals make up the remaining weight along with other nutrients.

The semisoft center of the bone contains *marrow*. Marrow is similar to a busy factory manufacturing red blood cells, which are necessary to adequately distribute oxygen throughout the body. In fact, each time the heart beats approximately 10% of the blood is pumped into the skeletal system!

Throughout a person's lifetime, bone continuously breaks down and rebuilds itself. Sometime after the age of 50, bone naturally begins to lose strength. This loss may progress due to decreased demands placed on the skeletal system.

The Spinal Column

What does the spinal column look like and what is its purpose? To visualize the spinal column imagine a tall building consisting of 33 floors. The blueprint of each floor resembles the level above and below. However, in the case of the spine, each floor may differ in size as some floors are designed to carrier heavier loads.

The components of the building, like the spinal column, hold the structure upright. Plus, the exterior of the building protects the contents, which in the case of the spine is the delicate spinal cord.

Looking at the spinal column's blueprint, each singular floor is called a *vertebra* (ver-tea-bra). When speaking of more than one floor, the correct term is *vertebrae* (ver-tea-bray). There are three types of vertebrae; *cervical* (sir-vick-all), *thoracic* (thor-a-sick), and *lumbar* (lum-bar).

In visualizing this imaginary 33-story building, one finds the top seven floors make up the cervical spine. The middle twelve floors of the building represent the thoracic spine. Looking down toward street level are the lumbar vertebral levels followed by the *sacrum* (say-crumb) and *coccyx* (cock-six), which might represent the basement levels of the building.

The *cervical* (sir-vick-all) *spine* begins at the base of the skull. There are seven vertebrae in this area with eight pairs of cervical nerves responsible for controlling the neck, arms, and upper body. This *vertebral* (ver-tea-brawl) group is sturdy enabling it to support the weight of the head. The amount of stress placed on these vertebrae varies with movement.

Directly below the cervical region the *thoracic* (thor-a-sick) portion of the spine starts. There are 12 vertebrae and 12 pairs of ribs, as well as nerve roots that control the midsection of the body. The ribs form the chest wall and protect many internal organs.

The third part of the spine is the *lumbar* (lum-bar) *vertebrae*. There are normally five lumbar bones. However, some people have one less or one more. These vertebrae are the largest and strongest of the three regions (cervical, thoracic, and lumbar) because these carry the bulk of the body's weight. Five pairs of lumbar nerves manipulate the movement and sensory functions of the lower extremities.

After the last lumbar vertebra is a mass of five smaller bones, which are naturally fused together forming a triangle. This bone mass is named the *sacrum* (say-crumb). Below the sacrum is the *coccyx* (cock-six) or tailbone made up of four little bones fused together. (Refer to Illustration 2.1 on the following page.)

The sacrum and coccyx do not look like the other vertebrae. The pairs of nerve roots originating from this area are responsible for the action of the pelvic organs and buttock muscles. The sacrum and tailbone could be considered the basement and sub-basement of the building.

When the doctor discusses a specific vertebra, its location is abbreviated. The vertebrae are numbered from the top of the spinal column to the bottom. For example, C-3 is the third cervical vertebra. 'T' denotes thoracic and 'L' refers to lumbar. The sacrum is simply labeled S-1. The coccyx is not abbreviated or numbered.

ILLUSTRATION 2.1

ANTERIOR (FRONT) VIEW OF THE SPINAL COLUMN

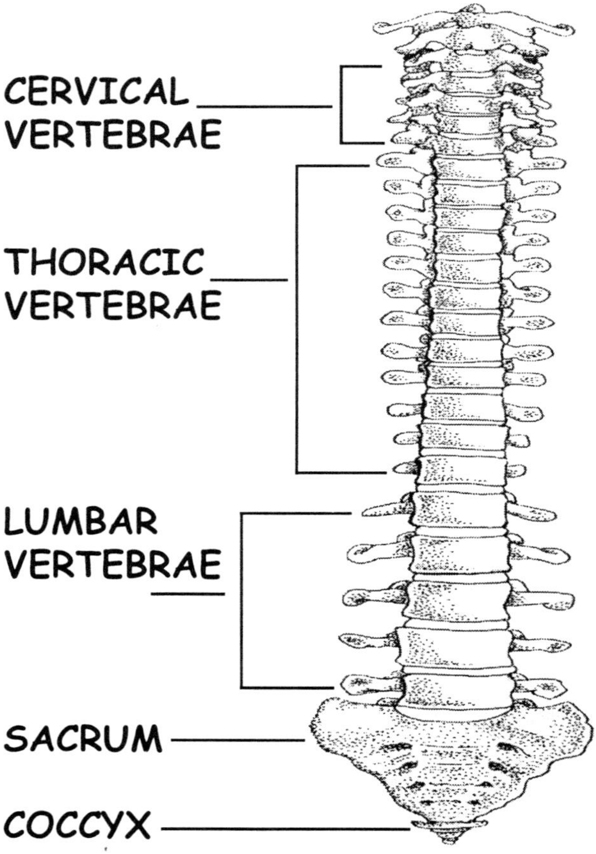

When a normal spine is viewed from the rear (posterior view) it appears vertically straight (Refer to Illustration 2.2 on page 13). However, when the spine is seen from the side (lateral view), three curves are revealed resembling a slight 'S' shape. (Refer to Illustration 2.3 on page 14.)

The spine curves gently at the cervical, thoracic, and lumbar regions. The curves serve as springs in a coil to distribute mechanical stress as the body moves.

In between each vertebra is a cushion-like *disc* also called an intervertebral disc (between the vertebrae). Collectively, these discs represent the spine's built-in system of shock absorbers. (Refer to Illustration 2.3B on page 15.)

Each vertebral disc is composed of a tough tire-like outer wall termed the *anulus* (ann-you-luss), which encases a soft gel-like center named the *nucleus pulposus* (new-clee-us pull-po-sus). (Refer to Illustration 2.4 on page 17.)

By the way, it is true that people are taller in the morning and shorter at night. While a person is lying down (i.e. sleeping) the discs absorb water and swell. However, once the person stands, placing pressure on the discs, some water is compressed out with movement. This is normal.

ILLUSTRATION 2.2

POSTERIOR VIEW OF THE SPINAL COLUMN

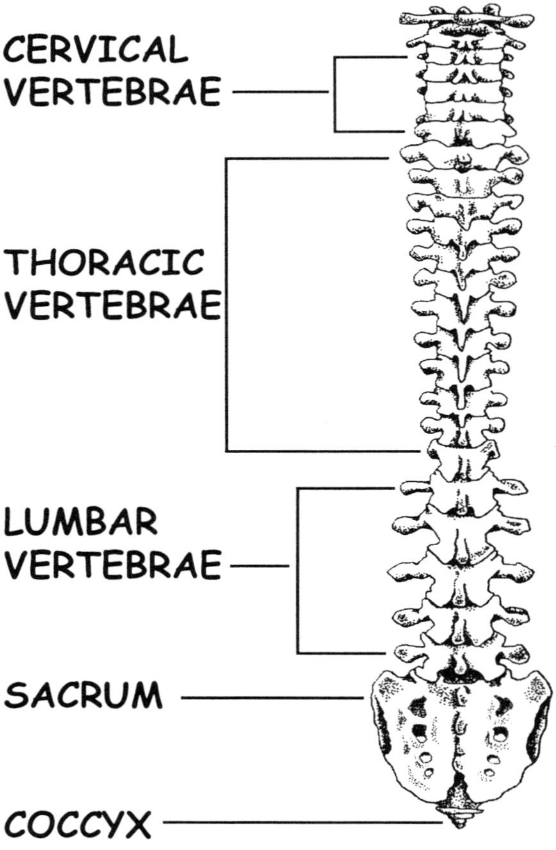

ILLUSTRATION 2.3

LATERAL VIEW OF THE SPINAL COLUMN

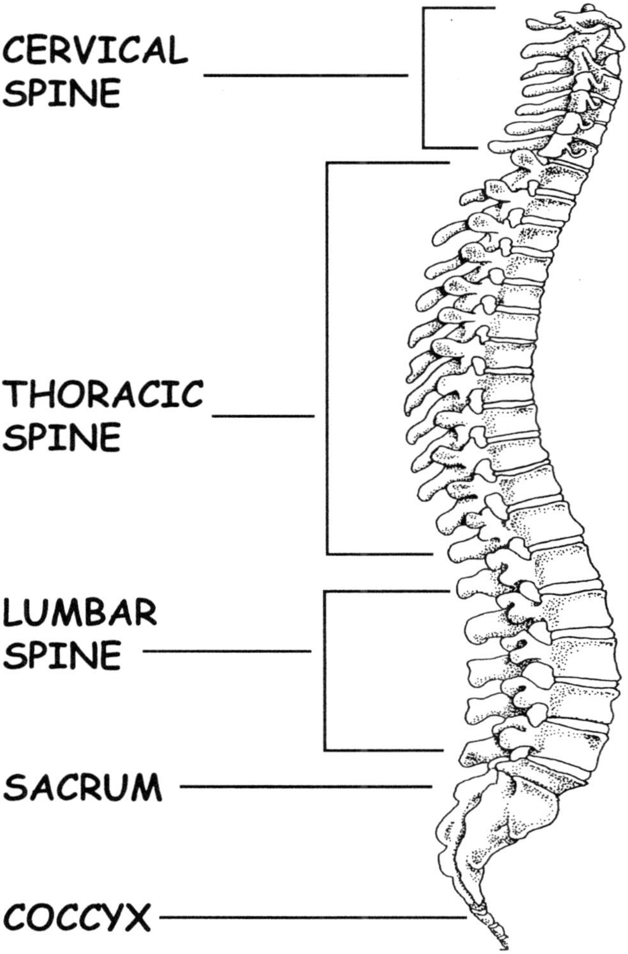

ILLUSTRATION 2.3B

SECTION OF LATERAL SPINE

Head
(Cervical)
↑
Body Front ← → Body Back
(Anterior) ↓ (Posterior)
Tail
(Coccyx)

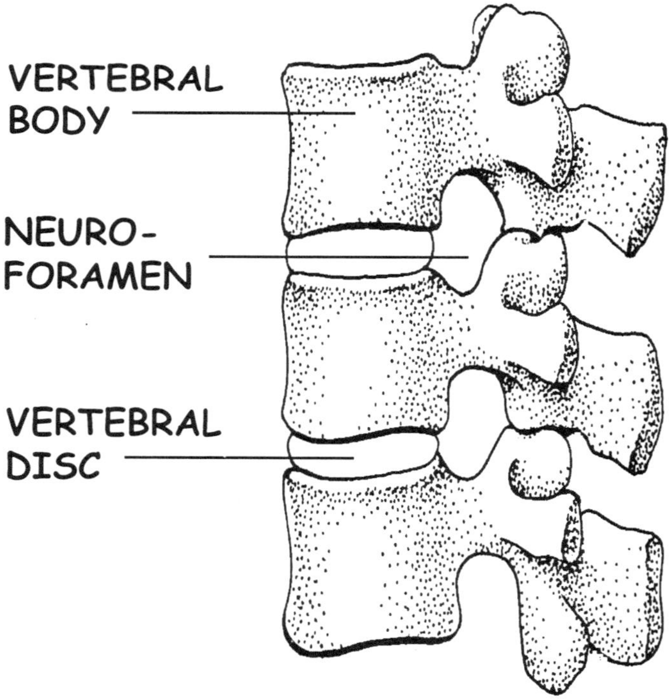

Unlike the 33-story building, the spine is designed to bend and turn. Along with the intervertebral discs, *facet joints* (fah-set joints) enable the spine to bend and twist. Each vertebra has two sets of facet joints.

One set of facet joints is located at the top and a corresponding set is at the bottom. Working like a hinge, the articulating surfaces of each facet joint are coated with smooth *cartilage* (car-till-edge) allowing friction free movement.

Although the facet joint bones fit snugly together, there is a lubrication system. The lubricating 'oil' is called *synovial fluid* (sin-no-vee-all) and resembles uncooked egg whites. This fluid also nourishes the cartilage tissues.

♦ ♦ ♦ ♦ ♦

The Spinal Cord

The spinal column is similar to a suit of armor that protects the delicate spinal cord. This is possible because inside the spinal column is a hollow canal. The spinal cord runs down through this space.

Three protective layers of membrane surround the spinal cord. These layers, similar to tubing, are the *dura mater* (dur-ah matter), or simply the 'dura', the *arachnoid* (ar-ack-noyd), and the *pia mater* (pea-ah matter). (Refer to Illustration 2.5 on page 19.)

ILLUSTRATION 2.4

ANATOMY OF A NORMAL VERTEBRAL DISC

-OVERHEAD VIEW-

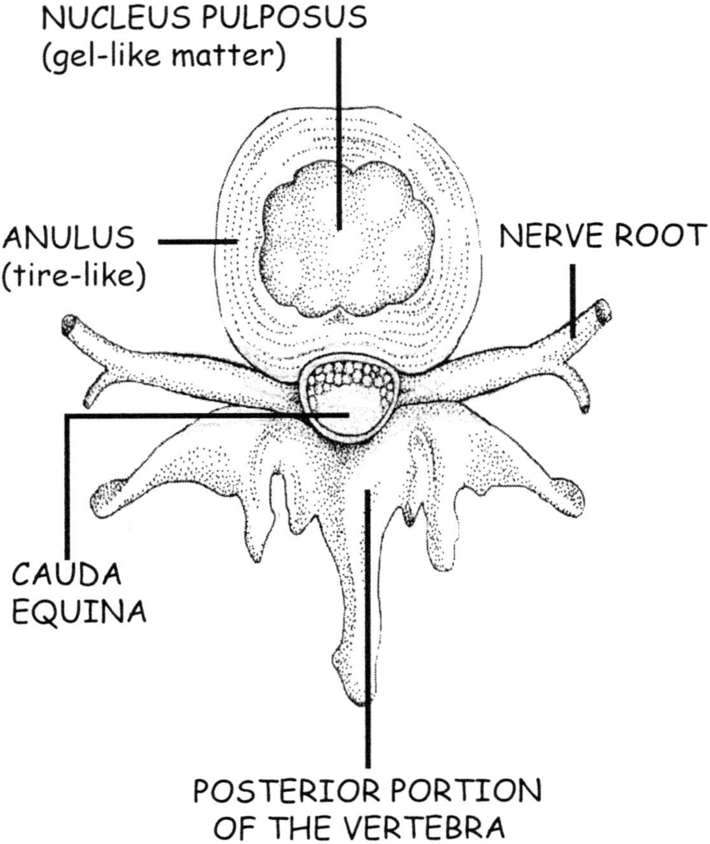

Cerebrospinal fluid (sir-ee-bro-spinal), created from plasma (derived from blood), flows in between each layer of the membranes. The fluid acts as a defensive cushion that protects the spinal cord, which is an organ central to the operation of the nervous system. (Refer to Illustration 2.5 on page 19.)

The spinal cord is about 18 inches long and begins at the base of the skull and ends just below the thoracic spine. At this point (the first lumbar vertebra) the spinal cord begins to resemble the tail of a horse (medically termed *cauda equina* (caw-dah e-queen-ah). The *hairs* of the symbolic horse tail are in reality the nerves (also called *rootlets*) that descend from the spinal cord above. (Refer to Illustrations 2.6 and 2.7 on pages 20 and 21.)

Between each vertebra, on both the left and right sides, a window is formed termed the *neuroforamen* (nur-row for-aye-men). The nerve roots slip through these windows and spread into the body like tree branches. (Refer to Illustration 2.3B on page 15.)

Not only do thousands of nerves send and receive signals from the brain to interior structures, but special nerves connect to the skin. *Dermatomes* (durma-tomes) are specific areas of skin controlled by nerve endings. Each dermatome originates from a single spinal nerve. In Latin, *derma* denotes 'skin' and *tome* refers to 'a section'. Illustration 2.8 on page 22 denotes the layers of dermatomes, some are labeled.

♦ ♦ ♦ ♦ ♦

ILLUSTRATION 2.5

INTERIOR VIEW OF THE SPINAL CORD

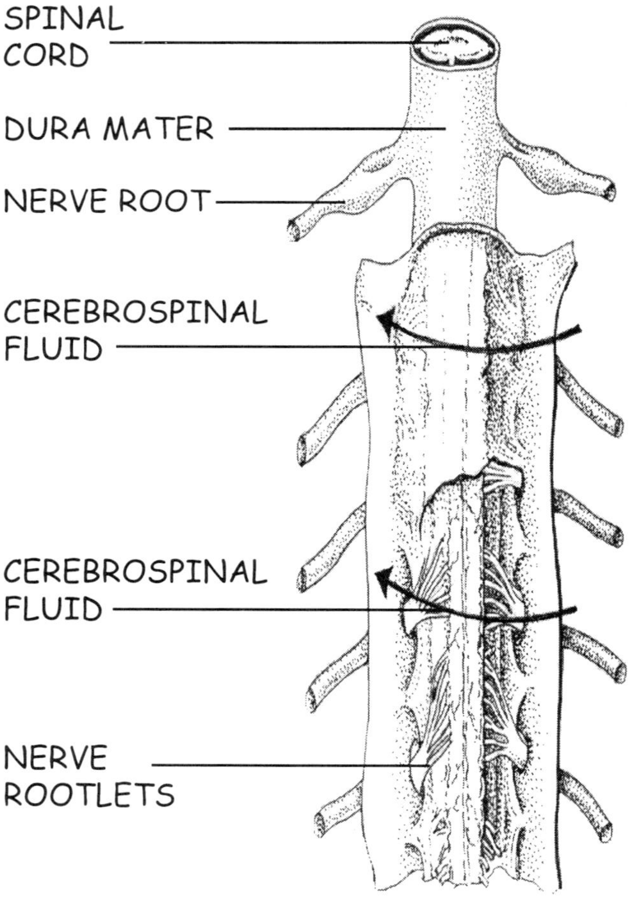

ILLUSTRATION 2.6

LATERAL VIEW OF THE SPINAL CORD

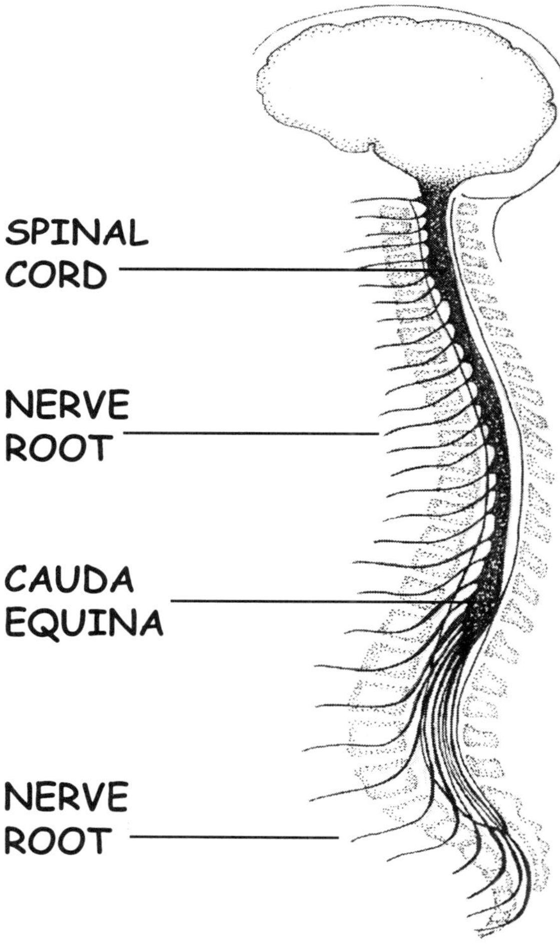

ILLUSTRATION 2.7

POSTERIOR VIEW OF THE SPINAL CORD

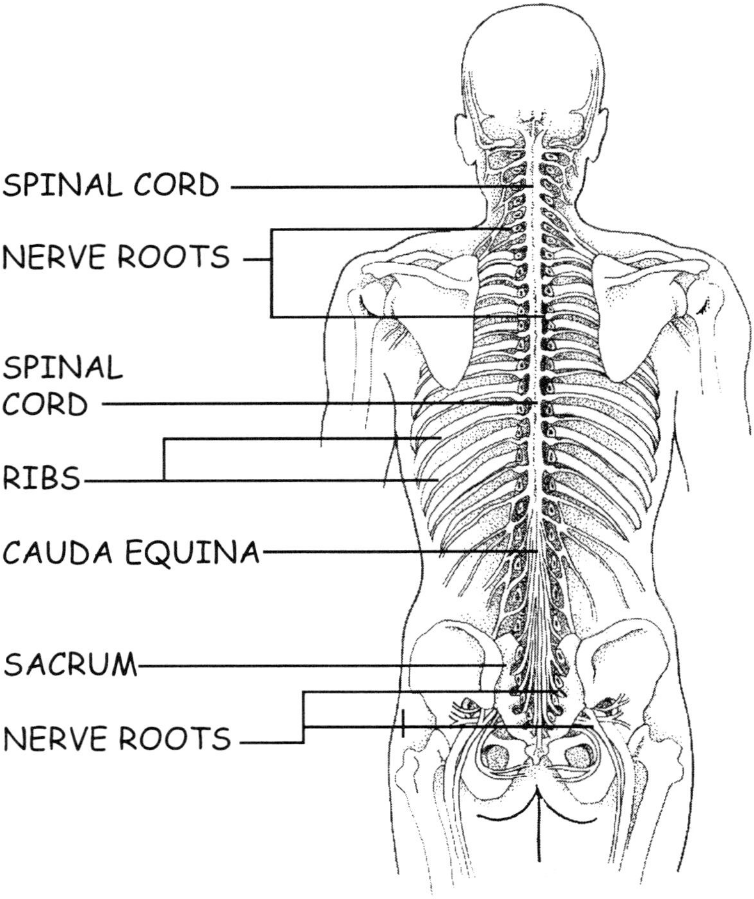

ILLUSTRATION 2.8

DERMATOMES

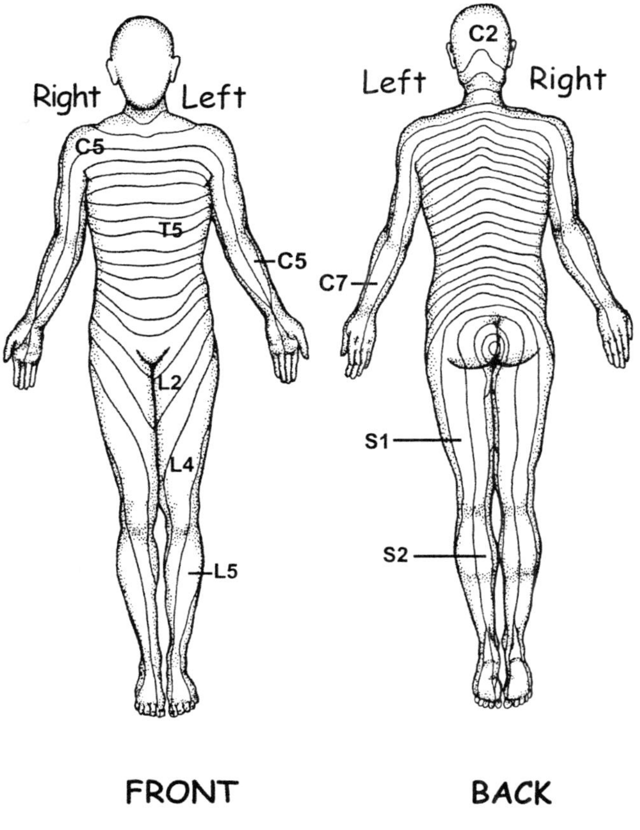

DERMATOMES OFTEN OVERLAP OTHERS. THERE ARE 8 CERVICAL, 12 THORACIC, 5 LUMBAR, AND 5 SACRAL. A FEW DERMATOME LOCATIONS ARE LABELED IN THE ABOVE DRAWINGS.

The Spinal Ligaments and Tendons

If the spinal column is designed to provide stability and protection, what holds bones together? *Ligaments*, similar to oversized rubber bands, criss-cross to hold the spinal column together. Ligaments are fibrous and strong tissue that connect bone, cartilage, and other structures supporting the spinal system. There are three major types of ligaments found in the spine.

... The *anterior longitudinal ligament* runs in the front (anterior) and vertically (longitudinal) attaching to the front of each vertebra.

... The *posterior longitudinal ligament* runs vertically behind (posterior) and inside the spinal canal from the brain to the tailbone.

... The third ligament, the *ligamentum flavum*, (lee-ga-men-tum flay-vum) acts as a protective hood over the dura mater. This ligament connects under the facet joints and forms a little curtain over the posterior opening between the vertebrae. This curtain can be pushed aside during surgery to allow the physician access to the spinal canal.

Sometimes the ligamentum flavum becomes enlarged and may create a blockage in an associated neuroforamen (window) resulting in nerve inflammation and pain. This problem may be remedied by surgically removing the offending tissue, which clogs the window and irritates associated nerves.

These three ligament systems are joined by smaller ligaments that also attach to the vertebral bodies to further safeguard the spine against bending too far in any direction.

Tendons are also an integral part of the spine. These sturdy bands of tissue attach muscles to bones. Tendons vary in length, thickness, and elasticity.

♦ ♦ ♦ ♦ ♦

The Spinal Muscles

The spinal muscles are a very complex system responsible for manipulating thousands of intricate body movements. Consider the graceful movements of a ballerina as she dances. The spine, ligaments, tendons, and muscles respond simultaneously as though choreographed. (Refer to Illustration 2.9 on page 25.)

Each muscle is similar to an instrument in an orchestra where the brain is the master conductor. The conductor speaks to each instrument through the movement of his baton. Each swing of the conductor's baton could be compared to nerve impulses directing the activity of the muscle.

Muscle is the only type of body tissue that has the ability to contract. It actually becomes shorter and thicker at contraction. Some muscles work in pairs or as antagonists. This means when a muscle contracts, the opposing muscle relaxes.

ILLUSTRATION 2.9

POSTERIOR VIEW OF THE SPINE & MUSCLES

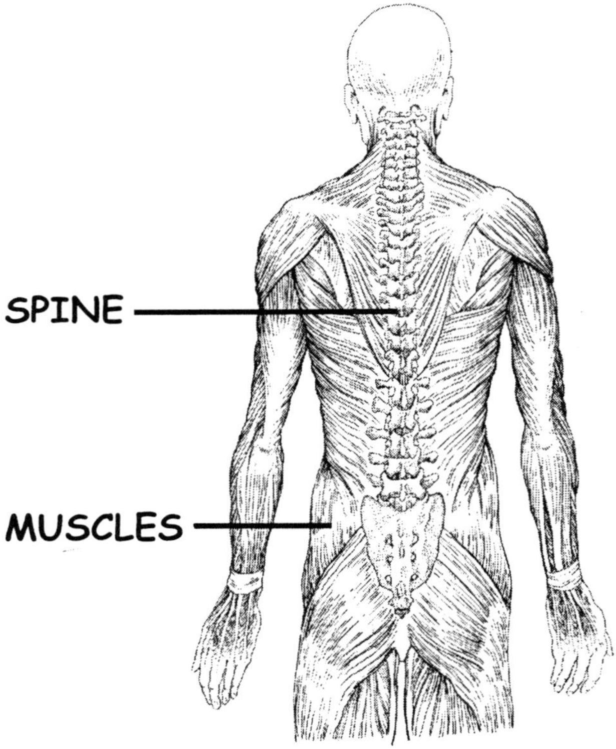

The muscles, along with the supporting system of ligaments, control the spine's ability to maintain balance and stability when a person stands or moves. Without the muscular system, the body would be motionless.

In Summary

After discussing the different aspects of the spine, it is easy to understand why such a complex structure would require special attention when injury occurs.

♦ ♦ ♦ ♦ ♦

Chapter 3

Consulting a Specialist and The Diagnosis

Let's say you have spent the last week in bed pampering your backache. At this point, you are beginning to doubt if the mattress possesses any curative powers.

You've taken your fair share of over-the-counter remedies and still have no significant improvement. Everyone in your family is tired of waiting on you and the dog no longer wishes to bring you your slippers. Perhaps it is time for some professional help.

♦ ♦ ♦ ♦ ♦

There are a number of disorders that can be responsible for inflicting back pain. Besides sore muscles and sprains, there are congenital and degenerative diseases, infections and, on rare occasions, tumors that can affect the bony and soft spinal tissues.

The spine is a compact environment occupied by bony structures, groups of muscles, ligaments, tendons, and nerves all living side by side. This arrangement could be compared to a neighborhood (spinal column) where the homes (vertebrae) have been built close together.

If one house catches on fire (i.e. pain from a compressed nerve), the nerve next door will likely be affected in some way. It is important to locate the source of the fire and extinguish it before the whole 'block' is on fire.

Some patients do not understand *why* they are in such agony. Their pain, when linked with apprehension, may promote feelings of anxiety and fear. Perhaps the patient does not know whom to turn to or whom to see about his or her disorder.

Depending upon the parameters of the patient's health insurance plan, the primary care physician may provide a referral if it is determined that more than routine care is necessary.

At this point, let's assume the patient has made an appointment to see a specialist. What is next? .... It might be a good idea to gather some information the physician needs prior to the office visit. The Checklist on the following page should be helpful.

☑ ✐ ✍

Pre-Appointment Checklist

☑ X-rays, MRIs, or other tests performed relevant to the current problem

✎ A few notes describing the type of pain, its location, and when the problem started

☑ Medical history including allergies, illnesses, family medical history, and prior surgeries

☑ Names and dosages of current medications

✍ List of questions for the physician

♦ ♦ ♦ ♦ ♦

The type and location of pain is very important to the physician in formulating the diagnosis. To help the patient describe his or her pain, a *Pain Diagram* is used. The patient is given the diagram to complete. (Refer to Illustration 3.1 on page 30.)

The pain diagram consists of two drawings; the front and the back of a human body specifying the left and right sides. The patient uses defined symbols to indicate areas of numbness, burning, aching, pins and needles, and/or stabbing types of pain.

ILLUSTRATION 3.1

PAIN DIAGRAM

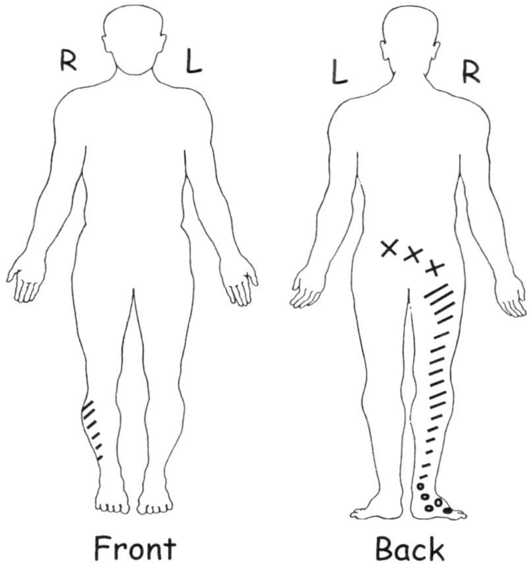

PAIN SCALE	PAIN TYPE
0 = Normal	Numbness
1	-------------------
2	Burning
3 = Low Pain	xxxxxxxxxxxxxx
4	Aching
5 = Moderate Pain	....
6	Stabbing
7	/////////////
8 = Intense Pain	Pins and
9	Needles
10 = Emergency	ooooooooooooo

Next, the patient rates each type of pain using a scale from zero to ten.

For example:

...Zero denotes normal feeling

...Five represents moderate discomfort

...Ten is equal to severe pain requiring emergency care

The patient incorporates this information onto each of the two drawings. A completed pain diagram enables the physician to visually identify the location, type, and intensity of the patient's pain.

♦ ♦ ♦ ♦ ♦

Next, is the physician's evaluation of the patient.

The evaluation consists of three basic steps:

#1 - The patient's medical history

#2 - The physical examination

#3 - Diagnostic tests, if needed

#1 - Reviewing Medical History

After the patient completes the paperwork, the physician's assistant or medical assistant guides the patient into an examination room. The assistant asks the patient questions necessary to complete his or her preliminary chart. Shortly thereafter, the physician arrives with the patient's chart and greets him or her.

The first part of the evaluation is a comfortable conversation between the doctor and the patient. The physician will ask the patient to clarify any unclear aspects of the medical history.

In addition, the doctor may ask auxiliary questions to gain a good understanding of the patient's past and current medical condition. Then the conversation will shift to a direct discussion about the patient's current disorder. Listed below are sample questions the physician might ask.

- .....When did the pain begin?
- .....Was its onset gradual or sudden?
- .....Does the pain radiate into the extremities?
- .....What was the patient doing when the pain started?
- .....What type of activity was the patient engaged in a day or two prior to the onset of pain?
- ......What activities aggravate the condition?

continued ...

◈......Is walking, standing, or sitting uncomfortable?

◈......Is the patient able to sleep?

◈......Has the patient been treated for this in the past?

◈......What therapy or medication has the patient tried?

Sometimes the physician is able to arrive at a preliminary diagnosis by carefully listening to the patient and analyzing what he or she says in terms of symptoms, past medical treatment, and family history. An accurate diagnosis is the key to a successful treatment plan.

♦ ♦ ♦ ♦ ♦

#2 -The Physical Examination

At this point, the patient may be asked to change into an examination gown. Depending on the patient's physical condition, the doctor may ask the patient to walk, stand, sit, and move the arms and/or legs. During this time, the doctor observes the patient's ability to move and range of motion.

Certain physical tests examine *bilateral response* (equal response on the left and right sides). Muscle strength is graded using pull and push maneuvers. Lower extremity deep tendon reflexes are found using a rubber hammer to gently tap each knee and ankle. Upper extremity deep tendon reflexes are tested at each bicep, elbow, and wrist. A mild jerking motion from the tapped extremity is a normal response.

The physician might perform a skin sensitivity test to gauge bilateral feeling in the extremities. Additionally, the symmetry of the extremities may be measured for size and compared left to right.

Areas of muscle tenderness are found during *palpation* (pal-pay-shun). Palpation simply means using the hands and fingers to place pressure on the skin and feel for what lies underneath. Skin temperature and color changes are also noted.

♦ ♦ ♦ ♦ ♦

#3 - Diagnostic Testing

During the first two steps, the physician is able to gather a lot of information regarding the patient's condition. At this point, the doctor has most likely determined a probable diagnosis. It is important for the patient to understand that tests are not done at random. Not every patient's problem will require an x-ray, CT scan, MRI, EMG, or lab tests.

Some disorders can be defined by clinical findings. The 'clinical findings' are clues the physician detects during the course of his examination, both verbal and physical. Most disorders, simple or complex, have distinguishing characteristics.

For instance, sciatica (sy-attic-ka) usually causes leg pain. The primary care physician may refer the patient to a spinal specialist. It is not unusual for a patient to ask the question *"Why examine my back when the pain is in my leg?"*

The answer is because the sciatic nerve runs downward from the spine into the leg. This type of pain is termed 'referred pain'. If the sciatic nerve is injured or compressed, chances are the foremost symptom will be leg pain.

Of course, the patient's medical history is very important in the diagnostic process, because certain pre-existing disorders, such as diabetes, could be responsible for a patient's pain resulting from a nerve problem. During the physical examination, the physician carefully notes the patient's responses.

When testing is ordered, it is done to detail the diagnosis. In other words, if a patient has the clinical symptoms for a herniated disc, an MRI or CT scan may be required to designate the exact location of the herniation. The MRI allows the physician to visualize the disorder, enabling him or her to make an accurate diagnosis leading to proper treatment recommendations.

Diagnostic tests are of great value. When the test results are combined with the findings from the first two steps, it is a *win-win* situation for both the physician and the patient. The physician is able to formulate an accurate diagnosis and offer the patient the best treatment options.

♦ ♦ ♦ ♦ ♦

Chapter 4

Diagnostic Tests

Fred has come to see his doctor today because he has a backache. The dialogue went something like this ...

Doctor:	"Well Fred, when did the pain start?"
Fred:	"Oh, a couple of hours after I played a game of golf."
Doctor:	"How many holes did you play?"
Fred:	"36 -- it was a great day for golf!"
Doctor:	"Um, when did you last play 36 holes?"
Fred:	"Oh, six or so months ago."

♦ ♦ ♦ ♦ ♦

After the doctor speaks to Fred a little longer and examines him, it appears the condition is not serious and is a simple soft tissue problem. In fact, Fred's backache did not even require an x-ray.

In this century, patients and doctors are truly fortunate to have available many reliable diagnostic tools. It is not uncommon for patients to ask about specific types of tests. The following topics have been addressed to answer many of these questions.

X-Ray

Probably one of the most common tests performed today is the x-ray. Just a little over 100 years ago, in 1895, Wilhelm Conrad Roentgen discovered the x-ray. This remarkable achievement radically changed the practice of medicine.

For the first time, physicians could see beyond the skin and other soft tissues to the skeletal system without autopsy. Roentgen did not entirely understand these unusual rays. He just knew he was able to see the bones in his hand. In fact he used the letter 'X' to describe the rays because in Algebra 'X' refers to an unknown.

When the spine is x-rayed, the beams pass through the soft tissues; skin, muscles, ligaments, tendons, and so on. However, when the beams meet bone, such as a vertebra, it stops, creating a white shadow on the film. Any bone abnormality could be reflected on the finished film. Shades of gray mirror the density of the tissues.

X-rays are still widely used today and are often referred to as a 'radiograph'. These tests are not performed at random. An x-ray would most likely be ordered when spine or extremity pain (i.e. a leg) is severe, perhaps following trauma from a motor vehicle accident or chronic progressive pain.

X-rays are used to rule out many problems that involve bone and some soft tissue disorders. In cases where x-rays prove inconclusive, additional tests may be performed, especially if something suspicious is detected.

CT Scan
(Computerized Axial Tomography)

In 1970, the CT Scan (CAT Scan) was developed. The CT scan evolved from Tomograms, which were multiple x-rays taken at different levels to check the depth of a defect. The advent of computers in medicine has enabled less exposure to radiation and shorter study times. With equipment refinements and use, the CT scan has become a viable adjunct to regular x-rays.

The CT scan utilizes multiple x-ray beams projected at many angles in conjunction with computer resources to create three-dimensional cross-sections of the exposed area(s).

Although some images may appear grainy, many levels of tissue are revealed in detail resembling slices. The slices are multiple small pictures from each layer of film.

MRI (Magnetic Resonance Imaging)

One of the most sensitive tools is the MRI. This medical miracle was first used on humans in 1971 and has become one of the most dynamic diagnostic tools. The equipment is made up of basically two magnets; one external and one internal.

The human body is composed of millions of negatively and positively charged atoms. In a sense, these atoms become similar to mini-magnets when they come into contact with electromagnetic waves produced by the MRI equipment. This data is combined using a computer, which is able to manipulate complex mathematical equations. When the calculations have been completed, the created image is transferred onto film.

MRIs are safer than CT scans because there is no exposure to radiation. The MRI represents the *gold standard* in imaging because of its ability to reveal the pathology of discs, nerves, and other soft spinal tissues in splendid detail.

For example, when the intervertebral discs are x-rayed, each disc usually appears as a pocket of air without detail. In contrast, an MRI provides a view of each disc in fine detail.

The MRI's ability to render pictures of soft tissues may help to identify soft tissues such as a disc or tumor. Additionally, contrast dye may be introduced intravenously to define an unclear image or highlight a particular area.

There are a few drawbacks to MRI. For example, take 100 normal people who appear to have nothing wrong with their spines and perform an MRI on each. The results may reveal that 20-25% of *asymptomatic* participants (without symptoms) will have a herniated or bulging disc, or some arthritic condition. These participants have no pain and their lives go on without interruption at that particular time. The disadvantage is the MRI results may create a false positive. This means the patient's test may reveal a disorder for which there are no corresponding clinical symptoms.

The point is ... the clinical symptoms must coincide with the test results. For example, in the author's practice, it is not uncommon for a patient to come into the office with a stack of MRI's and other reports indicating a herniated disc. However, the patient, a competitive tennis player, has no clinical symptoms (i.e. pain) for a herniated disc. In this particular case, to give the patient a serious diagnosis based simply on an MRI would be most regrettable.

This is why the MRI results *must* correlate with the patient's clinical symptoms for a specific disorder. In some cases, a disc can bulge and not cause any problem whatsoever. However, if leg pain is present and the MRI indicates a herniated disc in the area of the spine corresponding with the leg pain, it confirms the herniation as the source of the problem.

Some patients develop *claustrophobic* (claw-stro-foe-bick) feelings (fear of being in an enclosed place) inside the confines of the MRI imaging tube. These feelings may be avoided with medication prior to the test. Fortunately, more MRI facilities are utilizing open scanners, which are particularly patient-friendly to people who experience claustrophobia.

Since the MRI utilizes powerful magnets, patients with internal *ferromagnetic* (fair-oh-magnet-ick, a metallic iron) devices such as a pacemaker, metal cardiac valve, or metal in the area of the exam, cannot be scanned. Patients with these devices are referred for a CT scan.

Bone Scans

This test can be used to detect very fine stress fractures in bone, as well as arthritis, infections, or tumors. The patient is first injected with a liquid material that settles into the bone over a period of a few hours. During the test, the patient lies on the scanning table and a camera moves back and forth over the entire body.

An area of increased activity will light up brighter (termed a *hot spot* or *spot*) than other parts indicating a possible problem. This is a nonspecific test. When the results are *positive* (meaning something is abnormal), more specific investigation may be warranted.

Bone Density Scans

A Bone Density Scan is used to determine the compactness of bone. The computerized scanning equipment uses a low dose of radiation to measure the denseness of a hip or the spine. The test takes about 15 minutes and is easily administered. The results assist the physician in diagnosing men and women at risk for osteoporosis.

♦ ♦ ♦ ♦ ♦

SPECIALIZED TESTING for NERVE FUNCTION

The diagnostic tests discussed in the following sections are used to confirm or deny nerve involvement. For example, sciatic-like pain, which could radiate down into the leg, raises the question *"Is the pain coming directly from a leg muscle or is it a sign of nerve compression in the spine?"*

The following tests help the physician to answer questions of this nature.

Electromyography (EMG)

Electromyography (elec-tro-my-ah-graw-fee) is used to determine if muscle function is normal or abnormal. An EMG tests for the impulse coming from the brain and/or spinal cord. It follows that if the impulse is blocked somewhere in the spinal canal pathway, it may be delayed or diminished enroute to its final destination (i.e. muscle, skin, toe, finger tips). Thus, abnormal function could be indicative of nerve injury or muscle dysfunction.

Nerve Conduction Study (NCS)

A Nerve Conduction Study is a sensitive test usually done in conjunction with an EMG. The NCS stimulates the specific nerve(s) and records the nerve's ability to transmit the impulse. The study can reveal where the nerve is able or unable to function normally due to blockage.

Discography

Discography (diss-ah-graw-fee) is a type of x-ray used to view the intervertebral disc space and replicate symptoms for diagnostic purposes. During the test, the suspect disc(s) is (are) injected with a fluid that serves to illuminate it under x-ray. Abnormalities related to disc function or anatomical disorders may be determined from this test.

Laboratory Tests

The results from a simple blood test may determine if there is a possible infection, tumor, or other condition that can effect the spine. Sometimes these disorders are too small to be seen on a normal x-ray.

For example, a *urinalysis* (yur-in-al-eh-sis, testing the urine) might reveal kidney stones, which may cause severe back pain. A urinalysis may also find the by-products resulting from muscle breakdown created by dysfunction.

In Summary

The type of testing available today is truly remarkable, almost allowing the physician to pinpoint disease before its effects have become manifest. Osteoporosisis a classic example. In some cases, osteoporosis may be managed with medication, if detected early.

To learn more ... refer to the following chapter entitled Common Spinal Disorders.

♦ ♦ ♦ ♦ ♦

Chapter 5

Common Spinal Disorders

There are many types of back-related problems affecting the majority of the population in the United States. Although some conditions result from injury, several are related to a person's age, general health, and life-style. Whatever the cause, a spinal disorder may result from soft tissue injury, structural injury, or degenerative and/or congenital conditions.

◆ ◆ ◆ ◆ ◆

SOFT TISSUE INJURIES

Soft tissue injuries affect the non-bony and non-disc portions of the spine. Soft tissues are primarily the muscles, tendons, ligaments, and nerves. Unnecessary stress to the spine can be a contributing factor to injury involving soft spinal structures.

...The following numbers are relatively accurate *if* proper posture and body mechanics are used. Consider:

∗When a person lies flat on the back, *zero* pressure is exerted on the spine. As the person stands up the pressure climbs *three* times and while sitting *four* times!

∗When a medium weight box is lifted, the stressful force can rise to *five* times.

...But imagine how those numbers would escalate if improper movements were used! Consider:

∗An example of poor body mechanics is bending at the waist instead of at the knees to pick something lightweight up off the floor. This movement may wield as much as *10 times* the amount of unnecessary stress to the spine!

...Micro-trauma or mini-injuries to soft tissue may result from improper movement, especially when repeated. It is not surprising why so many people suffer from backache!

<u>Sprains and Strains</u> are part of this category. By definition, both conditions mean something has been stretched beyond its limits. For example, Dave has not shoveled snow since last winter and has decided to take care of his driveway after the first big storm. More than likely, Dave is going to suffer from sore and tender muscles. Why? Because Dave's muscles will be forced to perform beyond what he does on a routine basis.

When *muscle* becomes strained, the muscle has been forced to exceed its ability to work. Regular exercise can strengthen muscles and allow them to work harder longer, which is important considering muscles are the spine's work horses.

Sprains/strains can occur in a *ligament* or in a *tendon*. Ligaments attach bone to bone and tendons attach muscle to bone. A sprained ankle is a common example of a sprained ligament.

The bulk of the back is muscle. If enough force is applied to this soft tissue, injury can occur. This might occur during a motor vehicle accident when the body is suddenly thrown forward, backward, and/or sideways. Such forces can cause muscles, ligaments, and tendons to tear. When any of these soft tissues are injured, their respective repair factories switch into high gear to start the healing process.

The symptoms of sprains and strains are sudden, sharp, and persistent pain at the injury site, followed by swelling. Patients may first think a bone has broken.

If medical attention is sought, the attending physician will ask the patient several questions about the injury during the physical examination. If indicated, an x-ray will be ordered to rule out any abnormality. The physician may prescribe medication for pain, inflammation, and/or spasm during the healing phase. The patient's comfort is paramount.

Fortunately, the body has a great repair process, which quickly carries nutrition to the area. These injuries are usually self-healing in a two to three week period of time. However, recovery may be enhanced with physical therapy accompanied by a stretching program to prevent the formation of scar tissue, which may be debilitating.

Scar tissue is not normal tissue. For example, consider the scars left behind after a severe burn. In most cases, those scars are with the person for life, unless surgically removed.

In the case of muscles, ligaments, and tendons, the scar tissue may be trained by a physical therapist to mimic the function of the original tissue prior to injury. Where a ligament has torn, scar tissue can be used to aid in the healing process.

Muscle Spasms are common. Usually, muscles that have not been conditioned beforehand are not able to handle added demands.

When a muscle is overworked and/or overstretched its response is to go into spasm. The pain produced by spasm can be so severe the patient may think something is seriously wrong. This type of pain can be disabling, even causing deformed posture (i.e. bent to one side).

Whiplash is an intensive hyperextension injury that could cause micro-trauma to the soft tissue in the neck and/or upper back.

A car accident could force the head and neck to rapidly move forward, backward, and/or sideways. The muscles and/or ligaments attaching to the spine may be stretched beyond normal limits. The forceful and sudden action could cause micro-trauma or small tears in the muscles, ligaments, and/or tendons. Symptoms might include pain, burning sensations, and headaches.

If the patient is treated by a physician for whiplash, the patient may be given a soft cervical collar to wear, which lifts some of the skull's weight off tender neck and back tissues. The collar serves to immobilize and protect the cervical area during the initial healing stage.

In most cases, whiplash is self-limiting, which means it heals over a four to six week period of time. In some instances, whiplash may cause long lasting problems of a nonsurgical nature. In rare cases, whiplash may create a severe disorder requiring surgery.

◆ ◆ ◆ ◆ ◆

SPINAL NERVE INJURIES

Compressive Neuropathy (ner-awe-path-ee) occurs when nerves are compressed. The effects may be temporary or may permanently destroy nerves.

Foraminal stenosis (sten-oh-sis), which often occurs in the elderly, is an example of a compressive neuropathy. The nerves running through the spinal canal become trapped, compressed, and swollen. Foraminal stenosis can be extremely painful and debilitating.

Nerve compression may result when a disc slips, herniates, ruptures, or bulges. Nerves may become compressed or even displaced with the growth of bone spurs.

A compressive neuropathy may cause pain to radiate (ray-dee-ate) into the buttock (one or both), down the leg(s) as far as the knee(s), and can even be felt in the ankle(s) and foot (feet). Sensations of tingling, numbness, and weakness might accompany pain.

Sciatica (sy-attic-ka) is an example of a compressive neuropathy. Sciatica is a relatively common ailment named after the Sciatic Nerve.

The sciatic nerve is a collection of smaller nerves descending from the spine and joining together to resemble a cable. This nerve travels down through each buttock into the legs.

At certain points, such as in the posterior thighs, nerves branch off from the main sciatic cable. This is why sciatic pain may be felt in one or both thighs. (Refer to Illustration 5.1 on page 52.)

A direct blow to the sciatic nerve, which could occur during a fall, may result in injury to this nerve. The result from a sudden fall might initiate bleeding around the nerve(s) causing nerve compression and pain. Even coughing and sneezing could be considered as compression generators because these actions create pressure and may temporarily intensify pain.

When a disc or bone spur protrudes into the sciatic nerve cable, the problem may become severe. Even a bone spur could displace the sciatic nerve creating pain. Fortunately, there are conservative nonsurgical treatments that may be used to reduce the inflammation and associated pain, such as steroid injections and medication.

If the above interventions fail, and depending on the patient's symptomatology, surgery *may* be considered a treatment option. In some cases, a *laminotomy* (lamb-in-ott-toe-me) may be performed, which gives the surgeon greater access to the offending intervertebral disc.

<u>Peripheral Neuropathy</u> (per-if-fur-all ner-awe-path-ee) is another type of nerve disorder. This is a degenerative condition affecting the nerves branching into the body's extremities such as the arms, hands, legs, and feet. The disease causes the peripheral or distant parts of nerves to shrink.

ILLUSTRATION 5.1

SCIATIC NERVE

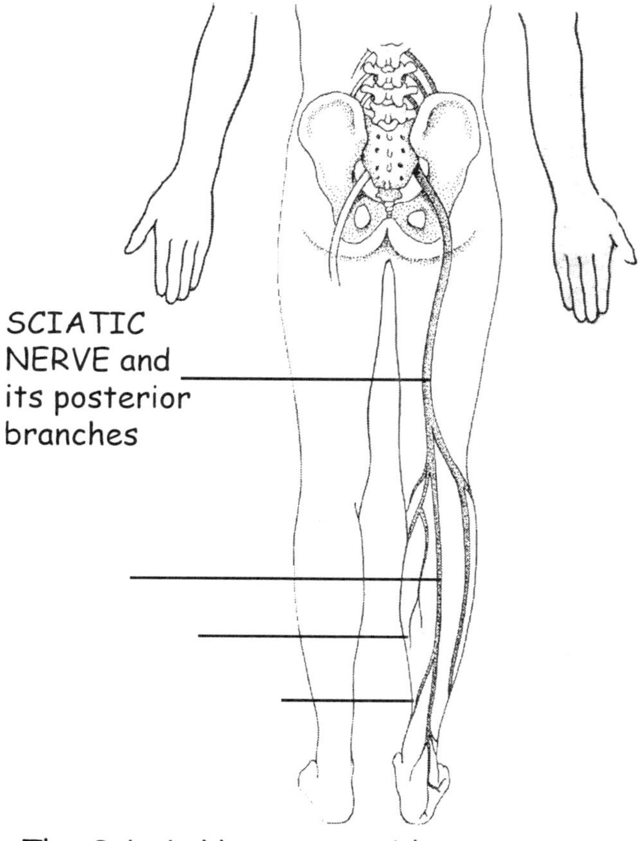

The Sciatic Nerve resembles a piece of cable exiting the spinal canal.

Sciatica, a common disorder, may result if this nerve structure is injured and/or compressed.

Eventually the nerves in the affected area may deteriorate. When the nerves can no longer carry impulses, sensory (feeling) and/or motor (movement) function(s) may be lost.

The patient may experience burning sensations, a feeling of pins and needles, an inability to feel the tips of the fingers or toes, and a weakness in grip and/or during walking.

The physician may be able to slow the effects of peripheral neuropathy with medication, but cannot cure or stop its progression.

Spinal Infections are rare and painful. Immediate medical attention is always warranted. If an infection is not detected and treated, the effected area swells and pain radiates into adjoining tissue. It may result in permanent injury.

A spinal infection may take root in the *epidural* (ep-eye-dur-all) cavity. This is a fatty area near a nerve and is a cozy home for an infection or abscess. These fatty areas are found in the cervical, thoracic, and lumbar spine. An MRI is usually performed to confirm the diagnosis.

Conservative treatment consists of intravenous or oral antibiotics combined with bed rest. If this approach is unsuccessful, then surgical interventions may be used to eradicate the infection and remove any affected spinal elements.

Spinal Meningitis (men-in-gi-tis) is a type of infection that causes inflammation of membranes in the brain and/or spinal cord. This is a serious disease that may require hospitalization. The patient is usually treated with intravenous or oral antibiotics combined with bed rest.

Some of the symptoms may include fever, weakness, pain radiating from the spine, muscle spasm, sensitivity to touch, decreased spinal flexibility, fatigue, sweating, and weight loss. When a child is affected, symptoms might include his or her refusal to stand or sit due to the pain. Increased backache may be a signal in older children and adults.

◆ ◆ ◆ ◆ ◆

STRUCTURAL INJURIES

In contrast to soft tissue injuries, structural refers to the bones and discs. Nerve roots may become irritated or damaged when an injury involves a vertebra or disc. Pain and/or weakness are symptoms that may accompany structural injuries.

Disorders affecting bony structures are explained in more detail on the following pages.

DISORDERS AFFECTING BONY STRUCTURES

<u>Spinal Fractures</u> are different from a broken arm or leg because these injuries may involve the spinal cord. Since the spinal column acts as the spinal cord's suit of armor, any damage to the column could place the spinal cord and its 31 pairs of nerve roots in danger.

Not only is a vertebral body vulnerable to breakage, but so are its attachments such as the facet joints, pars articularis, and spinous process. Damage to any of these bony components could jeopardize the integrity of the spinal cord and its nerve structures. (Refer to Illustration 5.2 on page 56.)

<u>Compression Fractures</u> of the spine are one of the more common injuries sustained by a vertebral structure. The vertebral body itself is the largest single unit of a vertebra. Its structural integrity is similar to a cardboard box.

Imagine a cardboard box; big and sturdy in appearance, but hollow on the inside. Now, let's say a great deal of pressure is placed on this box (vertebral body).

ILLUSTRATION 5.2

FRACTURE

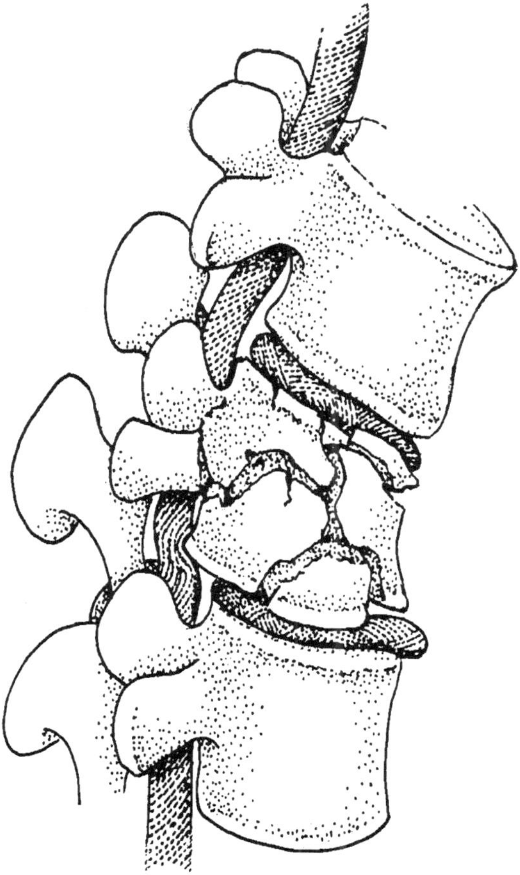

Perhaps a *hyperflexion injury* (hi-per-flex-shun) occurs. In this case, hyperflexion means the neck or low back is forced to bend too far forward or sideways. The result? A crushing effect causes the box (vertebral body) to resemble a wedge.

The amount of force delivered to each vertebra is shared directly with the surrounding spinal elements. It might be assumed the smaller cervical vertebrae would be more susceptible to injury simply based on size. Injury of this type generally does not occur often in the lumbar region, due to the size and density of the lumbar vertebrae.

Other fractures can occur from forces that cause the body to torque (twist). Even a direct blow to the spine can cause a fracture. Other parts of the vertebra such as the facet joints, or other bony processes, can break possibly causing dislocation of a vertebra and, perhaps, paralysis to some body part.

Although bone is a hard material, it can crack, split, or break away from the parent bone. Spinal fractures require immediate medical attention. An unstable fracture may be a serious condition causing one or more bone fragments to press against the spinal cord or nerves.

In osteoporosis (os-tea-oh-pour-oh-sis), a bone density disease, the effected bones weaken, become porous, and may become as delicate as fine porcelain. These bones are especially susceptible to breakage.

The type of fracture is determined by an x-ray. The treatment depends on the type of fracture and its location. Some fractures will require surgical intervention while others only need to be stabilized with bracing. One of the first steps is to stop movement to control and/or minimize damage.

When a vertebra breaks, the body's first response is to begin the healing process. Initially, a granular material termed a *callus* is formed at the fracture site. In addition, collagen, a protein is transported to the fracture site through the blood stream. Collagen assists in the mending or knitting process. After the new bone is sealed together with the old, it is hardened through a process termed calcification.

Years ago a patient with a broken back may have had to wear a plaster body cast. Fortunately, this is not the case today. Plastics have revolutionized the cast business. Most plastic casts are custom-fitted removable braces designed to be comfortable. Today, most spinal fractures may be more of an inconvenience than a tragedy.

Spondylolisthesis (spon-dill-oh-liss-thee-sis) is a fancy long term meaning one vertebra slips over another. Although this disease primarily effects the elderly as a degenerative disease, it may be congenital (present at birth) or discovered early in life. (Refer to Illustration 5.3 on page 60.)

Childhood spondylolisthesis can be caused when the pars articularis (par-z-are-tick-you-layer-es) does not fuse during early development. When these bony pieces do not grow together, a bony posterior weakness results in the vertebra.

Spondylolisthesis may result after injury or during overuse because the existing bony weakness lends the area susceptible to breakage. A physician whose speciality is the spine best deals with this condition.

Elderly spondylolisthesis may result when the stabilizing spinal structures begin to deteriorate. This occurs particularly in the lower back, which is responsible for carrying most of the body's weight. (Refer to Illustration 5.3 on page 60.)

Sometimes the spinal joints become arthritic and wear out, which may create spinal instability. As vertebrae lose their normal alignment, one vertebra might actually slip forward over the one below.

When a vertebra slips forward, the neuroforamen (window), where the nerves exit the spinal canal, may become closed causing nerve compression and sciatica. This condition is similar to spinal stenosis. (Refer to Illustration 5.11 on page 78.)

Pain and other symptoms may be alleviated with a surgical procedure termed a foraminotomy (four-ayemen-ott-toe-me). This procedure surgically increases the size of the neuroforamen and cleans away any debris that may clog the window.

ILLUSTRATION 5.3

SPONDYLOLISTHESIS (SLIP)

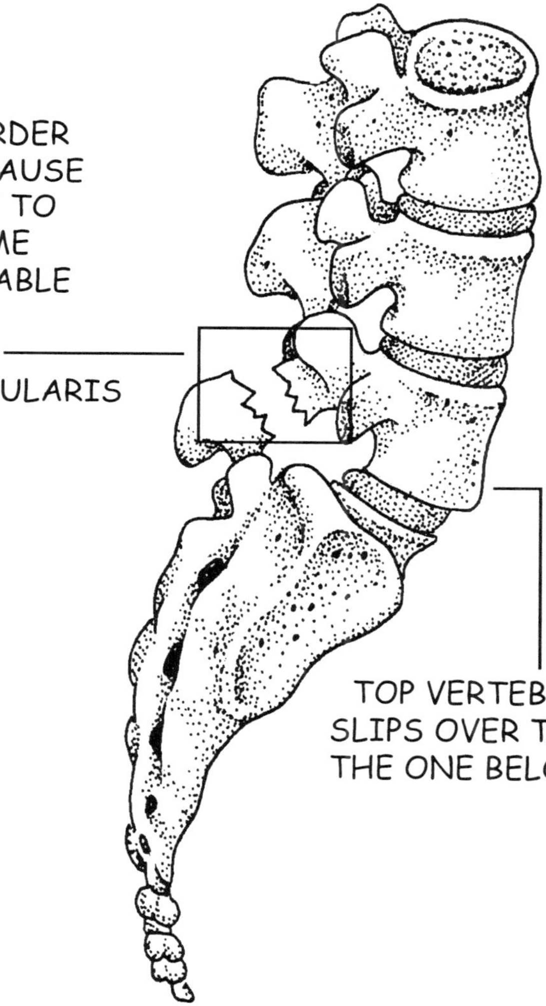

In most cases, spondylolisthesis can be treated nonsurgically with a course of physical therapy supplemented with steroid-anesthetic injections, prescriptions, and/or over-the-counter oral medications for inflammation and pain.

In a few instances conservative measures fail. Depending on the patient's symptoms, a surgical procedure termed a laminectomy (lamb-in-eck-toe-me, removal of bone) combined with spinal fusion may be necessary. Spinal fusion stabilizes the affected area(s) of the spine using hardware (rods, screws, plates) and bone grafting.

◆ ◆ ◆ ◆ ◆

TYPES OF SPINAL CURVATURE

Scoliosis (sko-lee-oh-sis) is a term taken from a Greek word meaning curvature. Throughout the 19th Century physicians thought poor posture was the primary cause of scoliosis. It is now known to be either congenital (present at birth) or developmental, and runs in families.

The disease causes the spine to curve laterally (to the side) usually in the shape of an 'S' or a 'C'. The curve can be mild to severe. (Refer to Illustration 5.4 on page 64.)

Kyphosis (ki-foe-sis) may occur due to poor posture early in life. Although kyphosis usually affects women, it can be found in men too. The excessive form of kyphosis may cause a hump to form in the shoulder blade area of the upper back.

Kyphosis may effect men and women with osteoporosis (os-tea-oh-pour-oh-sis). Although its onset may be more prevalent in women, it is found to a lesser extent in elderly men. (Refer to Illustration 5.5 on page 65.)

Lordosis (lor-doe-sis) can cause an extreme inward curve of the lower back. This condition is also referred to as 'swayback'. (Refer to Illustration 5.6 on page 66.)

Idiopathic Scoliosis
(id-dee-oh-path-ick sko-lee-oh-sis) is the childhood version of adult scoliosis. It is hereditary and primarily effects healthy young girls during their early teens. The physical signs may include uneven shoulders, one hip lower than the other, a rib hump when bending over at the waist, and leaning to one side.

Once maturity is reached, the disease may stabilize or slowly degenerate over time. Some adults have scoliosis, which probably began during their childhoods, but went unnoticed.

However, whatever the patient's age, the goal is to stabilize the spine to prevent additional curvature. Some patients with scoliosis are pain free and do not seek treatment until the deformity is noticeable. Unfortunately, at that point it may be too late to treat the disease.

To determine the degree of the curve, an x-ray is taken and the progression of the disease is monitored. In severe cases, the disease may cause the spine to rotate, resulting in narrowed spinal spacing on the opposite side of the body.

◆ ◆ ◆ ◆ ◆

ILLUSTRATION 5.4

SCOLIOSIS

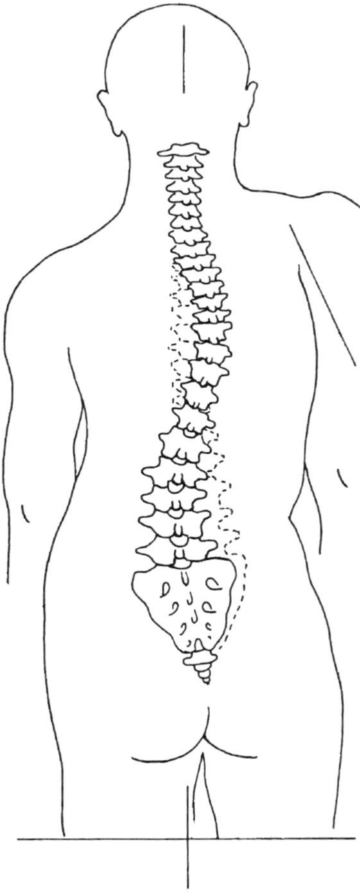

ILLUSTRATION 5.5

EXCESSIVE KYPHOSIS

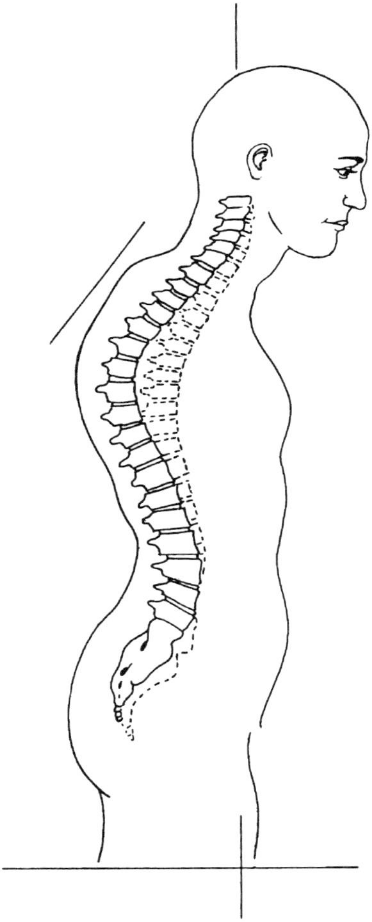

ILLUSTRATION 5.6

EXCESSIVE LORDOSIS

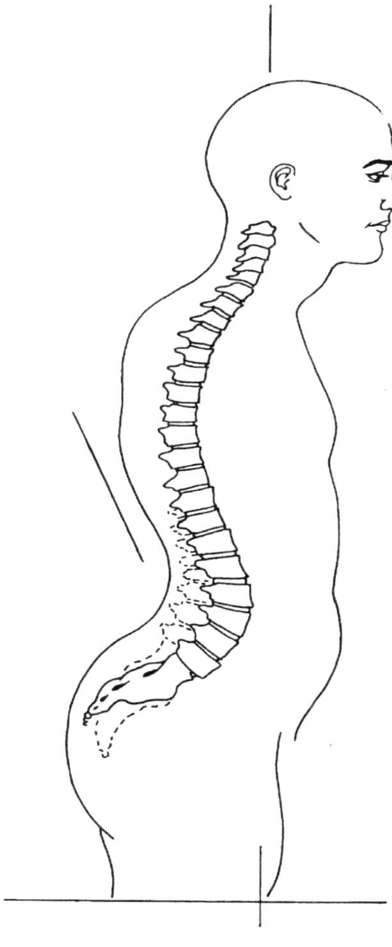

DISORDERS AFFECTING VERTEBRAL DISCS

In lay terms, a **Slipped Disc** may be used to refer to a **Ruptured Disc**. However, either term is better known medically as a **Herniated Disc** (her-knee-ate-it). (Refer to Illustration 5.7 on page 69.) Although the term 'slipped disc' is used, discs do not actually slip.

Each disc is sandwiched in between vertebrae supported by a system of ligaments designed to hold the spinal package together. Disc disorders are either *Contained* or *Non-Contained*.

An example of a *Contained Disc* disorder is a **Bulging Disc**. A disc that bulges does not break open; it keeps the nucleus pulposus 'contained' within the anulus. (Refer to Illustration 5.8 on page 70.)

A bulging disc could be compared to a volcano before it erupts and may be a precursor to an actual herniation. The disc protrudes into the spinal cavity without breaking open. The gel-like interior (nucleus pulposus) does not leak out. The disc remains intact, except a small bubble pops out attached to the disc.

A *Non-Contained Disc* is one that has either partially or completely broken open. This is termed a **Herniated** (her-knee-ate-it) or ruptured disc.

To illustrate, imagine a tube (anulus) of toothpaste (nucleus) placed under pressure. The pressure causes the toothpaste within the tube to move wherever it can. If any part of the tube is weak, pressure may cause the toothpaste to leak out.

When one or more discs herniate or rupture, the contents may spread toward nerves. The disc material has only one injurious place to go, back into the spinal canal where the nerve roots live.

Returning to the leaky tube of toothpaste, the disc's gel-like nucleus contains a chemical that irritates the nerves causing them to swell. After the chemical agent has done its job, the 'chemical blob' remains and continues to press on the irritated and swollen nerve(s).

To complicate matters, sometimes fragments from the anulus (the tire-like outer disc wall) break away from the parent disc and drift into the spinal canal. Once free fragments enter the spinal canal, they may travel up and down as though riding an elevator.

Depending on the type of injury and the condition of the discs, it is possible for more than one disc to slip, herniate, rupture, or bulge. Sometimes injury results in a combination of disc disorders.

◆ ◆ ◆ ◆ ◆

ILLUSTRATION 5.7

HERNIATED DISC

-OVERHEAD VIEW-

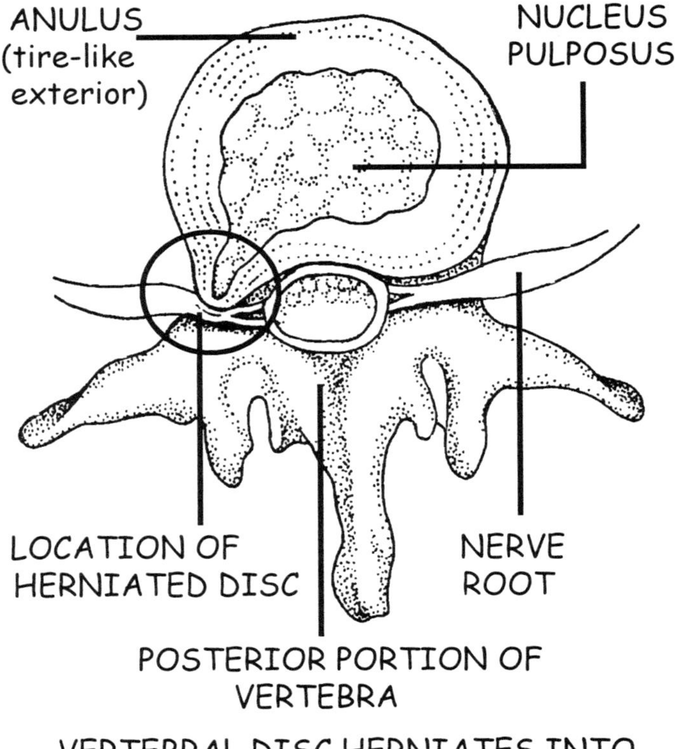

VERTEBRAL DISC HERNIATES INTO NERVE ROOT. NUCLEUS BREAKING THROUGH ANULUS.

ILLUSTRATION 5.8

BULGING DISC

-OVERHEAD VIEW-

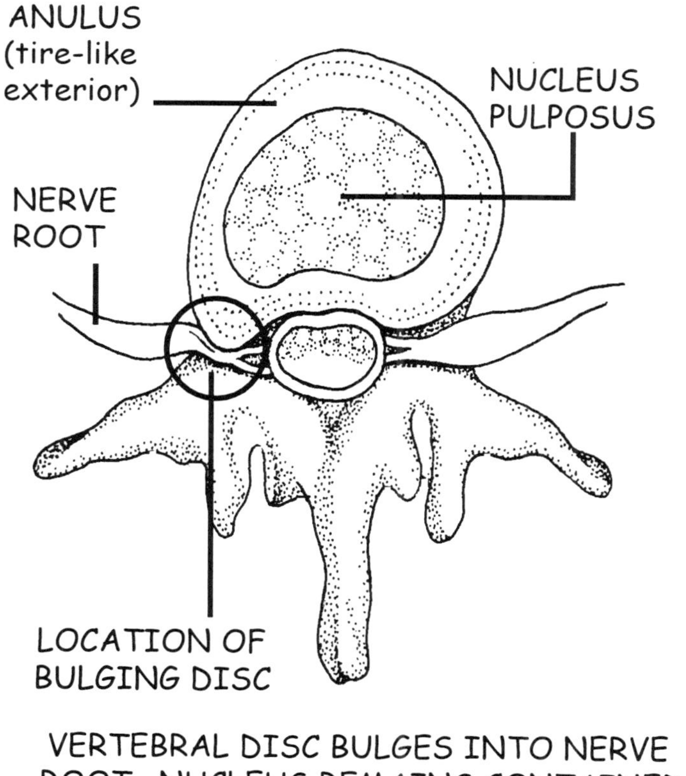

VERTEBRAL DISC BULGES INTO NERVE ROOT. NUCLEUS REMAINS CONTAINED WITHIN ANULUS.

DEGENERATIVE and/or CONGENITAL DISORDERS

Degenerative disorders are sometimes due to the process of normal aging and/or wear and tear. Just like mechanical devices, human bodies are subject to wear and tear from use. However, unlike machinery, the human body has the ability to heal or attempt to repair a problem.

At birth, the structural integrity of a person's spine, heart, lungs or any other organ system is at its peak for development through the years. During mid-life, early microscopic changes begin to appear that indicate the spine is aging. The spine does not deteriorate just because it ages. Wear and tear also play important roles.

Ailments such as arthritis, spinal stenosis, or osteoporosis do not develop overnight. Degenerative diseases may take many years to develop. These disorders may be associated with past injuries, abuse, body structure, or congenital problems.

Arthritis (arth-rye-tis) affects approximately 80% of people over the age of 55 in the United States. Injury, a weakened immune system, and/or heredity can trigger the onset of arthritis. Although there are hundreds of types of arthritis, the symptoms are similar: inflammation, joint pain, and a progressive deterioration of joint surfaces over time.

The joints may actually lose their normal contour, excessive amounts of fluid may build up inside the joint along with floating pieces of debris. This disease may be found in any of the spine's joints, those parts which enable the body to bend and twist.

Part of the problem may be the body's response to arthritis, which is to manufacture extra bone to stop joint movement. The extra bone is called a bony overgrowth or bone spurs. (Refer to Illustration 5.9 on the following page.)

In medical terminology, the extra bone is called *osteophytes* (os-tea-oh-fights). Osteophytes may be found in areas affected by arthritis such as disc or joint spaces where cartilage has deteriorated.

The body's production of osteophytes is really a futile attempt to stop the motion of the arthritic joint and deal with the degenerative process. It never completely works. The evidence of bony deposits can be found on an x-ray.

Since the facet joints are in close proximity to the neuroforamen through which the nerve roots exit, the arthritic bone spurs may cause nerve impingement. Sensory symptoms include pain, numbness, burning, and pins and needles in the extremities below the affected nerve. Motor symptoms (muscle) include muscle spasm, cramping, weakness, and/or loss of muscular control of a body part.

ILLUSTRATION 5.9

BONE SPURS or
BONY OVERGROWTHS

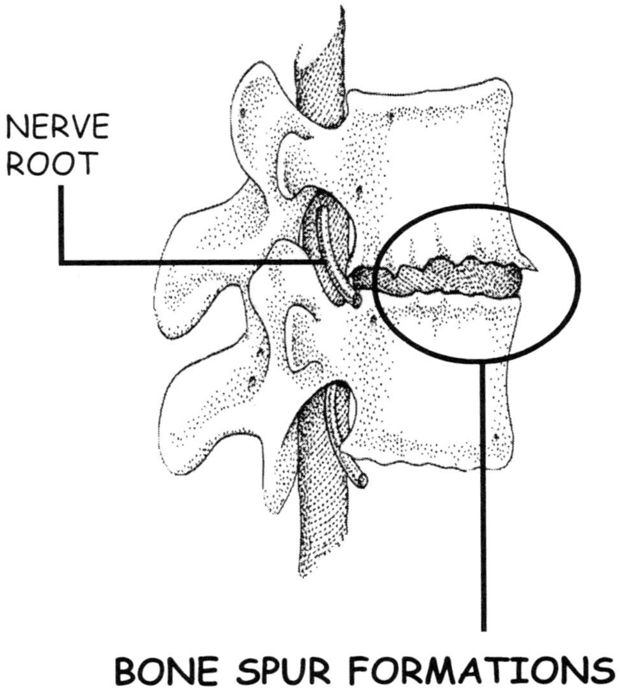

<u>Osteoarthritis</u> (os-tea-oh-arth-rye-tis) is the degenerative form of arthritis. Osteoarthritis is a progressive joint disease associated with aging. Many elderly people have some degree of osteoarthritis. It might be found in the knees, hips, or any other joint.

In the spine, osteoarthritis can affect the facet joints, which enable the body to bend and twist. As these joints deteriorate, cartilage may become inflamed and start to fray like a well used rag. The fraying process may cause pieces of cartilage to break away from the joint surfaces. The cartilage fragments might begin to float in the joint's lubricating fluid.

As the joints are stripped of their cartilage, the once smooth, slick surfaces designed for friction-free movement are lost. Joint bones may begin to rub together creating friction while trying to work. The nerve structures in the joint become sensitized, irritated, and may result in inflammation and pain.

Osteoarthritis may trigger the formation of osteophytes (os-tea-oh-fights). As previously mentioned, these bony spurs are the body's way of dealing with the disease.

In the spine, the bony spurs may cause disc space to narrow. When this happens, the associated vertebral disc may collapse, compromising its integrity. (Refer to Illustration 5.10 on the following page.)

ILLUSTRATION 5.10

OSTEOARTHRITIS

-LATERAL VIEW-

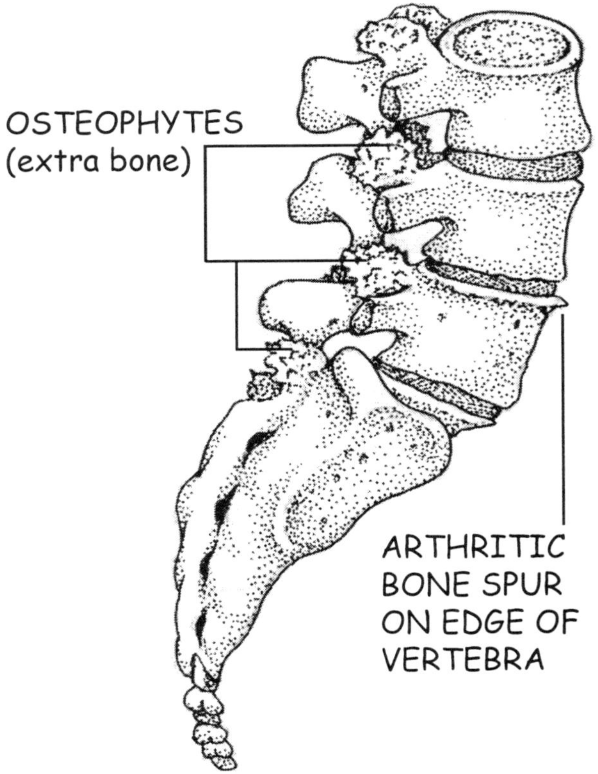

Rheumatoid Arthritis (RA) (room-a-toyed arth-rye-tis) is a progressive form of arthritis that can be painfully destructive. This disorder may cause the interior tissue of joints to swell and thicken. Over time, the affected joint(s) disintegrate, resulting in deformity. RA may appear during early middle age and is more common in women than men.

The symptoms may include fatigue, weakness, a poor appetite, fever, and anemia. Upon rising, joints are usually stiff, swollen, and tender. Medication is available to relieve the pain and to reduce inflammation, but a key is regular exercise to keep joints moving and functioning. Passive forms of physical therapy may be helpful to increase joint mobility.

Ankylosis (an-key-low-sis) is a progressive spinal disease that may cause the spine to gradually lose its flexibility and stiffen. It may be found to affect patients with arthritis and/or osteoarthritis.

Spinal Stenosis (sten-oh-sis) is a narrowing of the spinal canal and/or neuroforamen (windows) where the nerves exit the spinal canal. This disorder is associated with aging. Some people are predisposed to spinal stenosis genetically or it may be due to congenital problems. The disease can be easily explained by translating its meaning from Greek. *Spinal* denotes the spine and *stenosis* means the narrowing of a normally larger opening.

When the neuroforamen (windows) are partially or completely closed and/or clogged with debris, the spinal nerves become compressed and/or trapped. The symptoms of spinal stenosis may include numbness, weakness, burning sensations, tingling, and pins and needles in the involved extremity, such as the leg. (Refer to Illustration 5.11 on page 78.)

Spinal stenosis could be compared to wearing a pair of shoes that are a half size too small. The feet (nerves) react to the pressure by swelling (nerve inflammation), which makes the shoe even tighter. The pain (nerve compression) from wearing the small shoes can make walking difficult or impossible.

Patients with spinal stenosis have found the pain may ease when bending forward or sitting. This may happen because bending forward creates more vertebral space, which may temporarily relieve nerve compression.

Although spinal stenosis may affect any part of the spine, it seems to be more prevalent in the lumbar region. Pain may be felt in the buttocks, thighs, and/or calves when walking and/or standing.

Cervical spinal stenosis can affect the upper extremities and back. If severe enough, it could affect everything from the neck down.

ILLUSTRATION 5.11

SPINAL STENOSIS

A 'window' is used to illustrate the neuroforamen and the effects of spinal stenosis on the nerve roots.

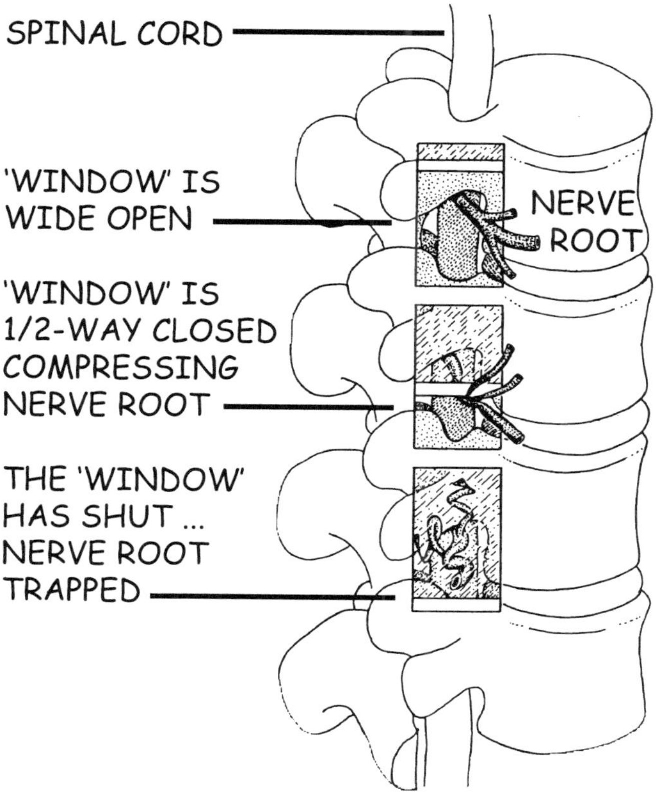

The patient's symptoms for spinal stenosis are often confirmed by either a CT scan or MRI. If absolutely necessary, a surgical procedure termed a foraminotomy (for-aye-men-ott-toe-me) can be performed, which enlarges the size of the window to help relieve nerve compression.

<u>Foraminal Stenosis</u> (for-aye-men-al sten-oh-sis) is associated with spinal stenosis, but is singled out because it primarily effects one or more vertebral foramen (window).

Normally, nerve roots have enough room to easily slip through the foramen. However, with age and disease, the windows (neuroforamen) may become clogged with debris. The nerves can become trapped and compressed.

The symptoms of foraminal stenosis may include numbness, weakness, burning sensations, tingling, and pins and needles in the involved extremity, such as the leg. Not every stenosis is critical, but if spinal stenosis is ignored, nerves may die, which could result in a loss of function. The functional loss could involve the ability to feel (sensory) and/or move (motor).

If conservative forms of treatment are unsuccessful, surgery is an option. The procedure termed a foraminotomy (for-aye-men-ott-toe-me) is discussed in Chapter 9.

Degenerative Disc Disease affects the vertebral discs. As each disc is placed under constant pressure during spinal flexion and extension, the discs absorb the stress created by movement. With age and motion, some disc wear and tear will naturally occur.

When the spine is x-rayed, the spaces between the vertebrae may appear narrowed indicative of degenerative disc disease. Discs that have become thin, or that have collapsed, can cause the vertebral space to narrow.

In addition, loss of disc moisture is simply one of many biochemical changes associated with aging. A similar chemical change occurs as a tire ages. As the tire loses its resilence, its original form may be compromised. The disc may shrink in size, wrinkle and/or even crack. Pieces of the disc may break away (i.e. creating fragments) and cause nerve irritation.

This could cause vertebral structures to compress causing the neuroforamen (window) to be reduced in size. The compressed nerves react by swelling and signaling pain. (Refer to Illustration 5.12 on the following page.)

ILLUSTRATION 5.12

DEGENERATIVE DISC DISEASE

-LATERAL VIEW-

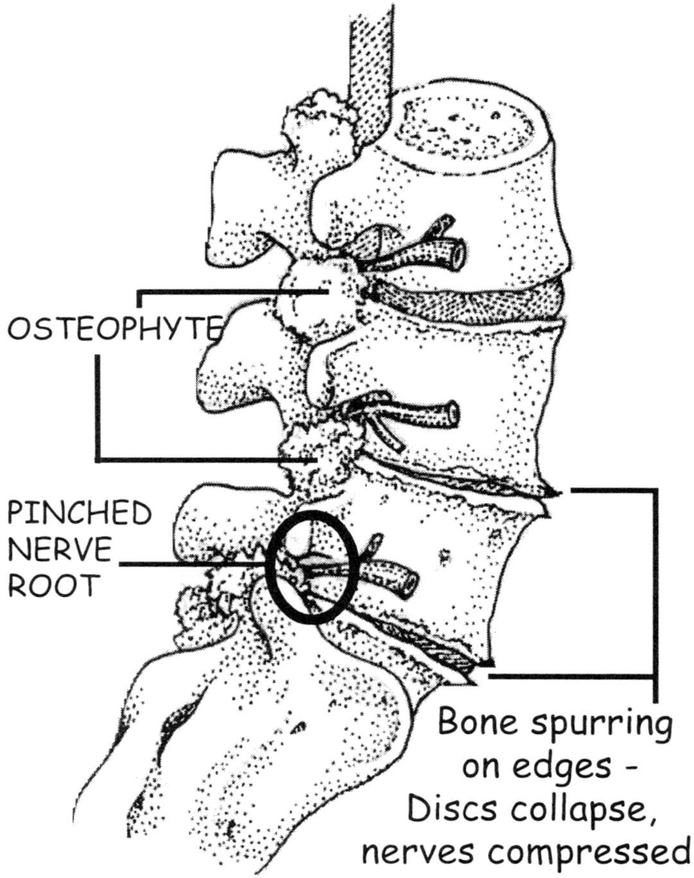

The neuroforamen could be compared to the brakes on a car. In this scenario, the vertebral discs are the brake pads, which act as a cushion between the foot pedal (top vertebral body) and the wheel (bottom vertebral body). With age, abuse, and/or wear and tear, the brake pads may become thin or may even disintegrate. What happens? The brakes squeal (pain) when used, or may not stop the car. Either way, the driver of the car will probably feel the effects of the faulty brakes.

People maintain their cars for dependability. A normal amount of wear and tear is expected and acceptable. The same is true of the spine. In most cases, as a person ages the physical demands placed on the body decrease. Today, through proper nutrition, consistent exercise, and prevention, the body can be in good shape at any age.

Osteoporosis (os-tea-oh-pour-oh-sis) is known as the *silent degenerative disease*. The disease is labeled *silent* because in the early stages, the patient may be symptom free. However, as the disease progresses, bones gradually begin to resemble a well used sponge: thin and porous (full of holes). Bone mass and density is lost. (Refer to Illustration 5.13 on page 85.)

Osteoporosis can affect any bone in the body, rendering bones extremely susceptible to fracture. It might be said that osteoporosis occurs when the body makes more calcium withdrawals than deposits, resulting in bankrupt bones.

When osteoporosis affects the spine, the symptoms may include chronic pain, loss of mobility, and an alteration of physical appearance. Patients may appear frail, bent over, and shorter.

Chronic pain may result from spinal muscles forced to take on the load once handled by the spine. Daily chores such as making the bed, removing a turkey from the oven, or even embracing a loved one could cause vertebrae to break.

Deformities may develop as the spinal bones become more porous and weakened. The breakdown of bone can eventually lead to compression and crush fractures, as well as a hunched back. Due to the loss of bone strength, spinal fractures may occur spontaneously without reason. The patient's weight alone can cause vertebrae to collapse. The associated nerves may become impinged, compressed, and/or destroyed.

As vertebrae collapse, height can be lost and internal organs may be forced out of their normal positions. Osteoporosis can be an insidious disease, which may eventually cause the patient's general health to deteriorate.

Although osteoporosis is a normal part of aging for both women *and* men, the key is to know the risks and reduce them. There are factors that accelerate the progression of the disease. Smoking, alcoholism, heavy use of laxatives, stress, diabetes, menopause, inactivity, and unhealthy dieting are examples.

Women smokers produce lower levels of estrogen. In addition, the smoking habit interferes with the absorption of calcium (Vitamin D), which is necessary for strong bones. Alcoholics, women or men, generally have less bone mass because calcium absorption is hindered.

The estrogen hormone is primarily responsible for maintaining sufficient calcium in the skeletal system. Stress can be an undermining factor because it may stimulate the *adrenal* (a-dree-nal) hormones, which could cause calcium to be passed during urination.

Women are more prone to osteoporosis than most men because, to begin with, a woman's bones are smaller, containing less mass. Estrogen levels are usually effected during the menopause. In addition, women have a longer life expectancy than men and therefore may have more time to develop the disease.

Fortunately, today there is a simple and painless test termed a *Bone Density Scan* (see page 42). This test measures the density of bone. If signs of osteoporosis are found, medication can be prescribed to help control the disease. Treatment is easily administered. The medication is available either orally (by pill) or in nasal spray form. Plus, the medication has proven beneficial in some cases by preventing spontaneous fracture(s).

ILLUSTRATION 5.13

VERTEBRAL BODY AFFECTED BY OSTEOPOROSIS

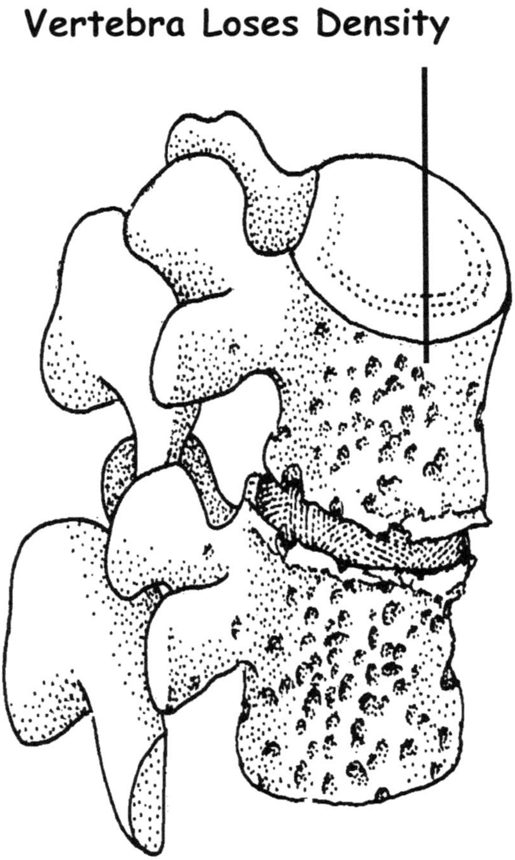

Since it takes years for bone to gain (or regain) strength, treatment is sometimes started when the patient is in the 60's. Later when the patient is older, the chances of a minor fall causing a broken hip or rib is minimized.

Besides medication, exercise is especially important at any age for several reasons. Physical activity can stimulate bones to become denser, good blood circulation nourishes bone, and healthy hormone levels can be maintained.

Weight bearing and resistance exercises, such as walking, build strong bones. However, before starting any exercise regimen, the reader should first check with a physician.

Spinal Tumors are rare. The physician will be primarily interested in determining the cause of the tumor and relieving any associated pain.

For example, if the patient's primary condition is breast or lung cancer, it is possible for the cancer to metastasize (ma-taz-ta-size, or spread) to the spine. The physician is always concerned if there is a past history of cancer coupled with a new history of back pain. The past and present histories may be related.

Tumors may occur in anyone without a history of disease. Fortunately, not all tumors are malignant.

◆ ◆ ◆ ◆ ◆

Chapter 6

Managing the Pain

PAIN (PAY-N) *N.*, 1. BODILY DISTRESS SUCH AS IN THE BACK, *SYN.* ACHE, ACUTE, AGONY, CHRONIC, DEBILITATING, ENDURABLE, STABBING SENSATION, SUDDEN SHARP TWINGE...

◆ ◆ ◆ ◆ ◆

Pain is a complex symptom that can affect the patient both physically and mentally. The intensity of physical pain may impede the patient's everyday activities such as driving the car to work, walking up or down a flight of stairs, sleeping, and so on. Prolonged inability to handle responsibilities could affect the patient's mental outlook.

From a functional point of view, nerve pathways, biochemical changes, and a patient's physiological and psychological makeup effect how pain is perceived. The side effects of pain often involve anxiety. Fear might result from simply not understanding "*Why am I in such agony? Is something dreadfully wrong?*".

Patient apprehension may build due to a loss of control over the situation and/or his or her self-treatment of pain. It is important for the physician to know if the patient has feelings of fear and anxiety. The physician will understand these feelings and knows that once fear begins to diminish, the pain may ease.

Pain control is a fundamental part of the care and treatment of back disorders. However, the core issue is the diagnosis (the cause of the pain). Whether the pain is acute (severe, but short-lived) or chronic (continuous), simply prescribing pain medication is not the answer to the problem.

One of the physician's objectives is to relieve the pain and keep the patient comfortable. The first step is to identify the source of the disorder and ascertain the severity of the patient's pain. As discussed in Chapter 3, this is determined from a review of the patient's medical history, pain diagram, physical examination, and test findings.

Anti-Inflammatory Drugs & Muscle Relaxants

Depending on the diagnosis, the first line of defense may include anti-inflammatory medication. Anti-inflammatory drugs reduce swelling and can help to relieve pain by simply alleviating pressure on the nerves.

Although many over-the-counter medications are available, the physician might prescribe a particular medication to suit the patient's individual needs. Sometimes anti-inflammatory and pain medication is supplemented with a muscle relaxant, which may help control spasms from muscles or nerves.

Narcotics

In some cases, to control pain of a more serious nature, narcotics might be used. These drugs are classified by government agencies as *controlled substances* due to their addictive potential. Narcotics may be administered orally or by injection and are used to control mild to severe levels of pain.

The doctor does not start off prescribing the strongest drug available. Instead, a less potent drug is usually tried first. The physician's goal is to prescribe the least amount of medication that will give the patient a reasonable level of comfort. Using medication as part of treatment is a way to help the patient through the acute pain phase, especially if there has been injury. It is the obligation of the prescribing physician to make certain he understands the cause of the patient's pain.

Once again, a proper diagnosis is essential. Physicians should not renew patient prescriptions without an accurate diagnosis.

Anti-Depressants

In some cases, anti-depressant drugs may be used in conjunction with other medication. These drugs are not only used to treat depression, but in some cases, may alleviate anxiety sometimes associated with pain.

Trigger Point Injections

A trigger point injection is a minimally invasive procedure. Medication is injected directly into the painful *spot* that appears to trigger the pain or spasm. The medication combines an anesthetic such as *Lidocaine* (lye-doe-cane), often used by dentists, and a steroid to decrease inflammation.

Nerve Blocks

In general, nerve blocks are a non-surgical approach to pain management. This treatment involves injecting a steroid-type medication around a nerve to decrease inflammation and reduce pain.

Epidurals

An epidural (ep-eye-dur-all) is a specific type of nerve block. Medication is injected into and around the spinal canal into the *epidural space*. The spinal nerves are located in this region.

Epidurals may be highly effective in managing pain from small disc herniations (neck and low back), milder forms of spinal stenosis, and arthritic conditions responsible for causing inflammation of the spinal nerve roots in the low back.

Post-Surgical Pain

Following a surgical procedure, some amount of post-operative pain should be expected. Some patients anticipate the onset of pain and may be concerned about its control. Many hospitals today use patient controlled analgesia (PCA) for their post-surgical patients.

PCA gives the individual patient control over the pain. This may allow the patient to rest more comfortably. The equipment consists of a pumping device with a finger control so the patient can self-dose pain medication through an intravenous line. Not only does PCA monitor the medication administered, but it helps to reduce the risk of over medicating a patient.

PCA use is gradually stepped down and replaced with oral medication to control pain while the patient is still in the hospital. Upon release, the patient may be sent home with similar oral pain relieving medication.

Moving forward ...

One of the goals in pain management is to help the patient to gain control over his or her discomfort. Once pain is in check, the patient may be able to move forward with a program of physical therapy.

Under the guidance of a professional physical therapist, the patient may be assisted a gradual return to a functional mode. For many patients, physical therapy is one of the keys to a successful recovery.

◆ ◆ ◆ ◆ ◆

Chapter 7

Physical Therapy

Physical therapy (PT) is a conservative form of treatment prescribed by a physician. It is a supervised and positive team effort. The orthopaedic surgeon or physician, physical therapist, and patient work together.

One of the physical therapist's goals is to help the patient with his or her activities of daily living (ADL's). These activities might include vacuuming, putting on socks, carrying groceries, getting in or out of the car, returning to tennis or golf, or resuming a walking program.

Initially, the patient might be asked to complete a simple questionnaire summarizing his or her ability to stand, walk and sit; the effect the ailment has on social life; the type, duration, and level of pain; as well as the ability to sleep, and care for him or herself.

Some patients may never have had any form of physical therapy in the past, and therefore do not understand the possible benefits.

This chapter is designed to answer many basic questions ... what is a Physical Therapist? ... why do some patients need PT? ... how many types of therapy are available? ... and so on. The following is presented in a Q&A format.

◇ What is a Physical Therapist?

A physical therapist is a medical professional who seeks to restore the patient's physical abilities to the fullest possible extent. Physical therapists receive extensive training during a four to six year specialized program.

◇ Why do some patients need physical therapy?

Physical therapy can be an important key to a patient's recovery. Under the guidance of a therapist, the patient gradually returns to a functional mode. He or she may be able to return to activities previously eliminated due to a painful back disorder. Various forms of therapy can help to reduce pain, improve flexibility, and regain strength.

A physical therapy program is individually designed to systematically restore the patient's functional abilities to the fullest possible extent. During physical therapy, patients can learn how to prevent re-injury and regain independence. The patient also learns how to manage at home with tasks such as household chores and personal hygiene.

◇ How does the physical therapist know what the doctor wants?

The physician gets the ball rolling by writing a prescription for physical therapy. The prescription tells the therapist the patient's diagnosis, the number of weeks, and times per week the patient is to receive therapy. The physician's order might include suggested treatment guidelines. However, the physical therapist is primarily responsible for making decisions about the design of a patient's therapy plan.

◇ What happens during the first therapy visit?

During the initial evaluation, the physical therapist and patient become acquainted. The therapist will review the patient's medical history to clarify information and answer the patient's questions.

Some patients have other functional problems (i.e. heart disease, diabetes, respiratory ailments) that must be taken into consideration when designing the physical therapy program. The therapist usually asks questions about the patient's level of pain, location, and duration.

Additionally, the therapist will want to know how and when the problem started, if its onset was gradual or sudden, what types of activities aggravate the condition, and so on.

During the initial evaluation, the physical therapist will observe the patient's posture and movement, noting any difficulties. For example, a patient with the disease scoliosis may present with a crooked appearance and an irregular *gait* (the patient's manner of walking).

Muscle weakness from a neurologic deficit may cause instability. The therapist will also evaluate muscle strength and the patient's range of motion (i.e. bending at the waist).

◇ Do all patients receive the same therapy?

No. After a careful evaluation, the physical therapist designs a treatment program to meet the patient's individual needs. The therapist manages the program, charting the patient's progress. Adjustments may be made to the program to help the patient accomplish goals.

◇ Are there different types of physical therapy?

Yes. Depending on the patient's needs, the therapy program might include ultrasound, electrical stimulation, myofascial release, flexibility and/or strengthening exercises.

♦ ♦ ♦ ♦ ♦

As stated, there are many types of physical therapy that may be combined for the patient's maximum benefit. Physical therapy includes, but is not limited to the following:

»Treatments given to the patient
»Movement & conditioning exercises
»Learning proper body mechanics

♦ ♦ ♦ ♦ ♦

TREATMENTS

Ultrasound is a common treatment that has been in use for over 40 years. Ultrasound uses high-frequency sound waves to promote deep warming of soft tissue, such as muscle. The warming affect promotes circulation and benefits healing. It can be used to treat muscle spasms and relax tight muscles.

Unlike a hot pack, ultrasound works without harming the skin (i.e. burning). The equipment controls set the speed of the sound waves. When fast moving sound waves hit the skin's surface, energy is transferred into surrounding soft tissue.

Electrical Stimulation, or 'stim' as it is often called, has proven benefits and is a widely accepted form of therapy. Physical therapists have used this modality for more than 15 years.

Stim forces a particular muscle, or muscle group, to contract and relax. During treatment, circulation can be *stimulated* to supply the target area with needed oxygen and nourishment during the repair process. Stim may help to enhance healing, alleviate swelling, and reduce pain.

But how does it work?

A pair of surface electrodes resembling beige-colored plastic rectangles is laid on the skin over the problem area. A pair of leads (insulated wires) connects the surface electrode patches to the equipment. The leads are like a phone line. Both ends of the line need to be plugged in for the system to operate.

The therapist sets the equipment controls to deliver the appropriate amount of stimulation for a prescribed period of time. The electrical current affects the nerve and muscle cells, which may either be at rest or reacting to the stimulus. The patient may experience a pleasant pulsating and/or an alternating on/off sensation.

<u>Treating With Heat</u> can be beneficial because it increases localized circulation, decreases stiffness, pain, and muscle spasm. Patients with early signs of arthritis may find substantial relief from their symptoms by taking warm baths or hot showers. This is best done early in the day to help to 'loosen-up' and alleviate the stiffness commonly associated with arthritis.

Another way to 'loosen-up' is in bed prior to getting up. A program of exercise designed to mobilize the hips and knees can be done. After getting out of bed, the patient may find the effects from the exercise can be enhanced by taking a warm bath or hot shower.

Physical therapists use canvas hot packs that swell when heated in water. The hot pack is wrapped in seven or eight layers of towels before it is laid or wrapped around the effected area. Unlike a regular heating pad that only delivers surface heat, a hot pack transfers moist heat. Moist heat allows greater heat penetration into soft tissue and stimulates localized circulation more than heat alone.

Myofascial Release is a *hands-on* modality used to improve circulation, decrease muscular tension, and promote increased range of motion. This treatment is a form of localized massage involving the underlying fascia. The fascia are sheets of fibrous tissue that encase muscles. During myofasical release, the fascia is manipulated by hand to systematically stretch the underlying tissue.

The therapy may decrease muscular tension and enhance healing. Scar tissue or tissue that is tight may be loosened using cross friction motion during massage therapy.

Hydrotherapy is probably one of the oldest therapeutic treatments. Hydrotherapy is similar to a whirlpool bath. Whirlpool tanks are available in sizes to even accommodate an entire body. During hydrotherapy both the water temperature and agitation can be controlled for maximum benefit.

Aquatic Exercise or water exercise may be especially beneficial to patients suffering from osteoarthritis. Not only does movement increase blood flow to affected joints, it can help to relieve stiffness. A pool also offers an anti-gravity environment, which may allow the patient to perform simple types of exercise without stressing painful joints.

For some patients, swimming is an excellent exercise to 'loosen-up' stiff joints and strengthen muscles. Patients should check with their physician or physical therapist before undertaking a pool regimen.

Treating With Ice can decrease pain by slowing the speed of nerve impulses. Inflammation, the body's vascular response to injury, may subside as cold interferes with circulation, reducing the temperature of tissue beneath the skin.

Cold packs, ice massage, and iced towels are usually recognized as first aid following trauma. However, treating with ice requires supervision by a physical therapist. This is especially necessary when treating an overworked body part.

♦ ♦ ♦ ♦ ♦

MOVEMENT and CONDITIONING

All exercise is done under the *supervision* of a physical therapist who can teach the patient how to move properly while pushing beyond pain thresholds.

Exercise Philosophy

Physical therapists want their patients to work in a *pain free* range. This does not necessarily mean exercise will be easy in the beginning. But remember ... *anything worthwhile is worth working for.*

Warming-Up

Generally, a whole body exercise, such as riding a stationary bike, is used to promote a systematic warm-up prior to therapy, followed by light stretching. The physical therapist will direct the patient during warm-up activities as outined in the patient's individualized program.

Stretching movements may help the patient to increase his or her flexibility. Resistive and strengthening exercises might be added to the patient's program. During this time, the patient will receive continued guidance and assistance from the physical therapist.

Some patients may not be able to move the affected area without assistance. In this case, the physical therapist manually moves the affected area (i.e. arm, knee) to help restore range of motion.

Patients, who begin without manual assistance, may experience temporary muscle soreness 24 to 48 hours after exercise. The *delayed onset of muscle soreness* is perfectly normal and may be expected. As regular exercise continues, the discomfort will slowly subside. Patients who are given a written/diagrammed home exercise program are wise to follow it regularly.

Always consult the therapist before starting or changing a physical therapy exercise program. If necessary, changes can be discussed with the patient's physician.

♦ ♦ ♦ ♦ ♦

PROPER BODY MECHANICS

The physical therapist will teach the patient how to move the body to prevent further injury during the recovery process. Many activities can be performed without the risk of injury (or further injury) if the patient is willing to maintain an adequate level of physical fitness, strive to reduce stress, and utilize proper body mechanics.

Proper Posture means maintaining the natural curve of the spine (neutral spine). Not only should proper posture be used when standing or sitting, but it should be incorporated into all activities of daily living thereby minimizing the amount of harmful stress the spine must bear. (Refer to Illustration 7.1 on the following page.)

ILLUSTRATION 7.1

PROPER POSTURE

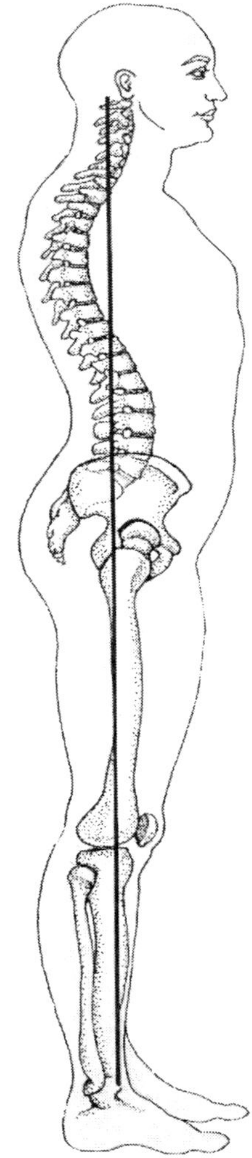

Proper posture is so important that it may be one of the first things the physical therapist teaches the patient. (Refer to Illustration 7.1 on the facing page.)

How is this done?

❖The shoulders should be held slightly back and level.

❖Each ear should line up with the shoulders.

❖The chin is slightly tucked and the pelvis is shifted forward so the hips are aligned with the ankles.

What does this look like?

❖Refer to Illustration 7.1 on the facing page.

❖The plumb line hangs from the ear lobe and drops down the middle of the arm to the ankle.

Why is this so important?

Poor posture and incorrect body mechanics are two of the leading causes of neck and back pain.

❖ ❖ ❖ ❖ ❖ ❖

The following suggestions may help the reader to maintain a neutral spine during activities.

Avoid Stressful Work Habits

Don't lean over the desk for prolonged periods of time.

- Don't sit too far from the work and/or with the back unsupported.

- Raise or lower the chair to the proper height so the knees are bent at a 90 degree angle.

- Keep the elbows bent at a 90 degree angle. The elbows may rest on the work surface.

- Don't bend or twist the neck to cradle the phone against the shoulder.

Standing ...

The feet should be placed slightly apart with the knees straight and chin tucked in to maintain a neutral spine. Do not stand in one position for a prolonged period of time, shift the weight from one foot to the other frequently. Using a footstool to elevate each foot from time to time may be helpful.

Sitting ...

Choose to sit in a chair that offers proper low back support. Don't slump in the chair! Try to keep the hips and trunk at a 90 degree angle.

Try to sit close to the work area and keep the feet flat on the floor or supported on an appropriate footrest.

continued ...

Think about keeping the chin tucked in while the head and shoulders are erect and balanced. Get up and/or change positions frequently. Don't become 'glued' to the seat. Get up and stretch!

Lifting Procedures ...

First take a look at the object to be moved. If it appears to be too heavy or cumbersome, find help! If there are obstacles in the way, move them *before* lifting the object.

Consider maintaining good posture and keep the head properly aligned. Try to get as close to the object as possible and bend at the knees.

Don't lift yet! Make sure the feet are slightly apart and flat on the floor. To turn, instead of twisting the body, pivot with the feet. This will help to provide a stable base of support.

Keep breathing and tighten the stomach muscles. Smoothly lift the object using the arms and legs ... *not the back!*

Carrying Procedures ...

First take a look at the object to be moved. If it appears to be too heavy or cumbersome, find help! Next, consider where the object is going. Are there obstacles along the way? If so, move them out of the pathway.

Depending on the shape of the object, try to hold it at the side and bottom while keeping it close to the body. Remember to keep the back straight. Carry the object with the elbows slightly bent.

An extra tip ... remember to carry a balanced amount of weight in each hand. For example, when carrying shopping bags or luggage, split the load in two.

Push or Pull?

Pushing is usually more efficient. Remember ... keep the back straight and use the knees to push. It is a good idea to stay as close to the object as possible. This may require repositioning the body from time to time.

Reaching Procedures ...

Consider the size, weight, and location of the object. Use a sturdy stool or ladder if necessary. Don't even think about standing on tiptoe!

Next, directly face the object and get as close to it as possible. One hand could be used for additional support. Try not to look overhead for prolonged periods of time. This could cause unnecessary stress to the neck.

Consider storing items that are used often within easy reach. This may mean rearranging shelves and/or closets.

Sleeping Tips ...

Even during times of rest, try to remember good posture. For example, the mattress should provide firm support for the spine, as well as the rest of the body.

Don't lie on the stomach. It is better to sleep on the back or side. When sleeping on the side, bend at the knees and hips. A comfortable option is to place a pillow between the knees.

Sleeping with a stack of pillows under the head may feel good, but doesn't benefit the natural curves of the spine. One moderately thick pillow should suffice.

A pillow here or there can really make lying down more comfortable. For example, to prevent sagging at the waist when lying on the side, try placing a pillow at the waist. And to help remove stress from the lower back, bend at the knees and slip a pillow underneath.

To Summarize ...

The therapies in this chapter represent many common and conservative types of treatment. The following chapter, Alternative Therapies, highlights a few of the more popular *alternatives* to conventional physical therapy.

♦ ♦ ♦ ♦ ♦

Chapter 8

Alternative Therapies

There are many types of alternative therapies originating from all over the world. In this chapter, Acupuncture, Biofeedback, Chiropractic, Reflexology, and Magnets will be discussed. Patients often have questions about these particular therapies.

Acupuncture (ack-you-pun-chure) was founded in China over 5,000 years ago and is based on the theory of Yin and Yang. When both are in balance, the body is said to be in a harmonious state.

The practice involves the insertion of special needles into specific parts of the body labeled acupoints. The needles are extremely thin with rounded tips that push the skin aside instead of cutting. There are over 1,000 acupoints. Most of these points are associated with the internal organs.

Today, acupuncture and Western medicine are frequently combined in treatment centers. It is not entirely understood how it works, but acupuncture has been proven to relieve pain.

Biofeedback is based on the theory that a patient can learn to consciously control pain to some degree.

Electronic leads (wires) are attached to the patient and connected to a myoelectric monitor. This monitoring device measures physiologic functions such as brain waves, temperature, heart rate, and muscle tension.

The patient is encouraged to relax using a technique such as imagery. As the patient becomes aware of physiological functions, he or she is trained to control those functions and thereby repress pain.

Chiropractic is based on the body's ability to heal itself through maintenance of the spinal column. It has been in use since 1895.

Prior to becoming a Doctor of Chiropractic, he or she learns manual manipulation skills and the interaction between nerves, muscles, and bones.

continued ...

A vertebral *subluxation* (sub-lux-aye-shun) occurs when the bones of the spine are not properly aligned. Chiropractic techniques are used to manually readjust the alignment of the spine.

Magnets can be used to treat specific body parts including the neck, and upper and lower back. These special magnets possess magnetic fields, which can enhance the flow of oxygen and nutrients deep into targeted tissue.

Reflexology is similar to acupuncture except needles are not used. Instead, the practitioner uses his or her fingers and thumbs to apply pressure to specific points on the patient's hands and feet that correspond to the ailment.

Practitioners of reflexology believe that the body's natural healing ability can be promoted by applying pressure to these points.

♦ ♦ ♦ ♦ ♦

Chapter 9

If All Else Fails ... Spinal Surgery

The Myth:
... the only solution a spine surgeon can offer is surgery ...

If you believe that, you might be interested to know that out of 100 patients seen with back problems, fewer than 5% generally require surgery. This means that an overwhelming 95% are treated using nonsurgical techniques.

If your problem falls into the 95% bracket, the first steps taken may include anti-inflammatory medication, an analgesic for pain control, physical therapy, and/or injections. If this traditional approach proves ineffective, and if the examination and findings warrant, then surgery *might* be considered an option.

In the category ... *fewer than 5%* requiring back surgery, some may arouse more concern. Notably, incapacitating back pain, inability to move the extremities, and/or leg pain associated with a loss of bowel or bladder control may be signs of progressive neurological deficit. In those cases, surgery may be the immediate course of action.

Another portion of the 5% may have unrelenting back and/or leg pain that cannot be controlled with injections or medication. The patient may have leg function, but may lack the ability to walk any distance thereby interfering with the ability to function on a daily basis.

Keep in mind that surgery is not the perfect answer or cure. Back surgery has its own risks and is very different from hip replacement or any other operation. Medical technology has provided well-functioning artificial hip joints, but spinal surgery does not share the same level of advancement. However, that is not to say the surgeon does not have any viable treatments to offer the patient.

At one time spinal surgery was reserved for the younger to mid-life population. Fortunately, attitudes have changed and current research shows that elderly patients can do quite nicely. The risks in spinal surgery may be well controlled and the success rate may be as high or higher than for younger population groups.

This may sound strange, but seniors are *sometimes* more motivated to get better than some younger people. Younger people may have more underlying problems such as those associated with family, stress, and depression. This does not mean that seniors do not share some of these problems, but they often have few difficulties.

This is interesting because modern research reveals the population as a whole is showing an increase in aging. Since the aging public is on the upswing, new progressive and degenerative spinal conditions will probably develop. Aging disorders include osteoarthritis, spinal stenosis, and degenerative disc disease. During the next 25 years, physicians will probably be dealing more with an expanding aging population. Many of the issues discussed in this chapter deal with surgical procedures affecting seniors in our society.

However, not every patient with an operable condition is a candidate for spinal surgery. Candidacy relates to the patient's general medical health. For example, someone with a cardiac disorder may be at a higher risk during any surgical procedure.

A person whose prior back surgery failed might be advised against an additional operation because one failure can sometimes lead to another. This might be attributed to predisposing factors such as smoking and/or diabetes.

If the patient is a smoker, he or she should stop at least one month prior to the operation. Nicotine can cause blood vessels to constrict slowing the circulation of blood. Good blood flow is essential for healing.

Without a healthy flow of blood, nourishment is not carried as quickly as needed. Additionally, bone simply does not grow or heal well when nicotine or any tobacco product is consumed. It is generally acknowledged that people who smoke are apt to have more spine problems.

Similar problems may be associated with other self-destructive habits such as excessive alcohol consumption, self-treatment for disorders using over-the-counter drugs, and/or mega vitamins as food supplements.

◆ ◆ ◆ ◆ ◆

The Goal in Spinal Surgery

The goal in spinal surgery is to restore the patient to his or her pre-disease/injury functional level as quickly as possible. This means improving the patient's symptoms, which usually relate to neck and/or arm, or back and/or leg pain. The success rates are very good in the majority of spinal surgical procedures.

Patient's Fears and Apprehension

For many patients, the thought of spinal surgery can be absolutely frightening. Fear or apprehension is a perfectly normal feeling. No one wants to have surgery of any kind if it can be avoided.

Fortunately, in most cases spinal surgery is not done on an emergency basis. Therefore, the patient and family members have time to discuss the issues concerning the procedure with their spinal surgeon and other physicians.

◆ ◆ ◆ ◆ ◆

THE STEPS LEADING TO SURGERY

The following *steps* will give the reader an idea of what to expect when surgery is recommended. However, keep in mind, if the patient does not want surgery, his or her decision is always respected.

Step #1 - When Surgery is Recommended

If conservative forms of treatment have failed and surgery is recommended, the surgeon may contact the patient's primary care physician. This might be done to obtain medical clearance from the patient's regular doctor. In other words, the surgeon speaks to the primary care physician about the patient's disorder and outlines his proposed surgical plan.

Step #2 - The Surgical Conference

In the author's practice, a patient whose condition warrants surgery will participate in a special conference with the surgeon and/or surgical assistant. The patient and family member(s) are invited to sit down with the surgeon and/or surgical assistant for a period of time longer than the usual office visit.

continued ...

During this surgical conference the patient's medical history and test findings may be reviewed. The surgeon explains in detail the nature of the disorder and how the surgery will be performed. The patient is encouraged to actively participate in the conference by asking questions. The surgeon explains any risks or possible complications that may be encountered during or after the procedure.

Some patients want to know if they can go home the same day of their procedure (i.e. same day surgery). Same day surgeries are procedures that may be defined as minimally invasive. Some types of surgery require a short hospital stay. The surgeon and/or surgical assistant will outline what to expect.

One common myth is that a long recuperative period in bed is necessary after back surgery. This simply is not true. In many cases the patient is up the next day walking. Even after a complex spinal procedure, the patient may be out of bed the following day, in a chair, and walking down the hall within two days.

The trend has definitely drifted away from confining patients to bed. In fact, rehab may be started the day following surgery to begin to restore function. Many patients are quite independent within a short period of time after surgery, even if the surgery was an elaborate procedure.

During the conference the patient will be asked to sign a document termed an *Informed Consent*. An informed consent outlines the type of procedure to be performed and includes the points discussed with the surgeon and/or surgical assistant. In most cases, the surgical outcomes are quite good with very little risk to the patient. However, since this is a sensitive area, it is best addressed with a clear plan in writing.

Additionally, from a psychological point of view, a well informed patient, who knows what to expect, may be less anxious about the upcoming surgery.

Step #3 - Hospital/Outpatient Pre-Registration

At some point prior to the surgery, the hospital or outpatient facility will call to schedule an appointment for the patient to pre-register. Pre-registration is a simple process. Depending on where the surgical procedure will be performed, either a hospital or outpatient facility staff member will verify the patient's name, address, social security number, and insurance information.

Step #4 - Pre-Operative Tests

Sometimes the pre-operative tests are done the same day the patient pre-registers. Or, the patient's primary care physician might administer the tests. The results of the tests are faxed to the hospital or outpatient facility.

The pre-operative tests usually include a chest x-ray, blood work-up, electrocardiogram, and urinalysis. The nurse will review the patient's past medical history, noting any allergies and medication taken on a daily basis.

Step #5 - Meeting an Anesthesiologist

If the pre-operative tests are done at the surgical facility (either hospital or outpatient facility), the patient might meet briefly with an *Anesthesiologist* (ann-es-thee-zee-all-oh-gist). During this meeting, if the patient has questions, the anesthesiologist will take time to answer each inquiry to the patient's satisfaction.

Modern *anesthetics* (ann-es-tha-ticks) are designed to keep the patient comfortable and pain free during surgery. ***Local anesthetics*** (locals) are injections near the procedure site. Locals work by blocking the pain signals sent to the brain. ***General anesthetics*** temporarily affect the nervous system by disabling nerve impulses. In other words, the patient is asleep and pain free. For open back procedures, general anesthetics are primarily used.

Step #6 - Pre-Operative Instructions

Before the patient leaves, the nurse writes out a list of pre-operative instructions to be followed the day before surgery. The instructions may include the time and place the patient should report for surgery, not to eat anything after midnight, and to take all daily medication the morning of the procedure.

Step #7 - The Day of Surgery

When the patient arrives at the facility, he or she is escorted by a nurse to a private room and instructed to change into a gown. Although the patient's belongings are kept in a safe place, it is best to leave jewelry and other valuables at home.

The nurse then reviews the medical information in the chart with the patient verifying his or her name, type of procedure to be performed, allergies, and other information. Then the nurse will start an IV (intravenous line) in one hand.

The IV line is used to inject medication directly into the blood stream. Shortly thereafter, the patient may be given a sedative. Sometimes patients become so relaxed they do not remember being wheeled into the operating room.

The operating suite is a sterile environment with large overhead lights above the operating table. During surgery the anesthesiologist monitors the patient's heart rate, blood pressure, and level of sedation.

Surgery is a team effort with the surgeon taking the lead. The surgical assistant and nurses support the surgeon and anesthesiologist as needed.

When the surgery is over, the surgeon and/or surgical assistant go into the waiting room to speak with the patient's family about the outcome of the procedure.

After surgery the patient is moved into the *recovery room*. In the recovery room, nurses monitor the patient's vital signs. Although still sleepy, the patient may then be moved into a regular hospital room. Patients who have had *same day surgery* (done on an outpatient basis) are released to go home *only* after they are fully awake and stable.

Step #8 - The Day After Surgery

Depending on the type of surgery, walking may be encouraged the next day. Although the patient might require assistance, movement keeps the blood in motion and enhances healing.

Physical therapy may then be added to help the patient build strength and flexibility. Post-operative physical therapy usually continues on an outpatient basis for a prescribed period of time.

Post-operative pain is relative. Some patients, who have lived with pain for years, recognize the difference between acute (severe, but short-lived) and chronic (continuous) pain.

However, after some procedures, the patient may only experience mild discomfort. In general, most people think of surgical pain as acute. It is important for patients to understand there will be some level of post-operative pain or discomfort.

Step #9 - Going Home

Whether the patient is released the same day or spends a couple of days in the hospital, he or she will be sent home with written instructions. If the surgeon has written prescriptions, these will be given to the patient along with the home instructions. It is always important to follow these instructions.

◆ ◆ ◆ ◆ ◆

COMMON SPINAL SURGICAL PROCEDURES

There are several new techniques enabling spinal surgery to be done on an outpatient basis. *Percutaneous* (per-cue-tain-ee-us) or *endoscopic* (en-doe-sca-pic) procedures are minimally invasive, which usually allow the patient to go home the evening of the surgery.

More invasive surgical procedures may require two to four days of hospitalization. After surgery, physical therapy may be incorporated into the treatment plan to increase mobility, build strength, and enhance flexibility.

After an invasive procedure, a nurse may be assigned to come to the patient's home to check all aspects of the care. Some patients may recuperate in an extended care or inpatient facility, similar to a hospital where recovery is closely monitored.

◆ ◆ ◆ ◆ ◆

PERCUTANEOUS
and
LASER PROCEDURES
(Minimally Invasive)

Percutaneous (per-cue-tain-ee-us) surgical procedures are performed through a small hole made into the patient's skin instead of an incision. This is similar to *endoscopic* (en-doe-sca-pic) surgery, a technique used in some abdominal surgeries.

Through this small hole a *cannula* (can-you-la, a small metal tube) is passed into the affected area. This type of surgery falls into the category of minimally invasive, enabling the patient to recover quickly.

Small hand instruments and/or a laser device can be passed through the cannula into the surgical site. Many of these procedures are done using *fluoroscopic* (floor-oh-sca-pic) *guidance*. This means the surgeon can see the location of the instruments on a video monitor while he performs the operation.

A *laser* (lay-zer) might be used if a disc herniation is small. The surgeon starts by inserting the laser through the cannula. Once into the disc, the center of the disc may be vaporized. The disc should then retract centrally toward the hole created by the laser.

In other words, the herniated disc pressing on the nerve root pulls back toward the center of the disc. After the pressure on the nerve has been alleviated, the pain may diminish. After the surgery is completed, the small hole is covered with a bandage.

◆ ◆ ◆ ◆ ◆

DISCECTOMY and MICRODISCECTOMY

Both terms mean the surgical removal of part or most of a vertebral disc. The difference between *discectomy* (dis-eck-toe-me) and *microdiscectomy* (micro-dis-eck-toe-me) is the latter procedure uses a microscope during surgery.

Either procedure can be used when appropriate to remove herniated or ruptured discs. The advantage to microdiscectomy is the incision and instruments used are smaller in size. Any procedure that is less invasive enables the patient to recover more quickly.

◆ ◆ ◆ ◆ ◆

LAMINOTOMY and LAMINECTOMY

The easiest way to remember the difference between these two terms is that the suffix *ectomy* (eck-toe-me) means *to remove.*

For example, an appendectomy (ap-pend-eck-toe-me) is the removal of the appendix. Both terms ... laminotomy and laminectomy, relate to the *lamina* (lamb-in-ah), or thin bony layer, which is part of each vertebra. This thin layer may partially obstruct the surgeon's view of a disc through the spinal canal.

<u>Laminotomy</u> (lamb-in-ah-toe-me) means the *partial* removal of the lamina (thin bony plate) to reveal the underlying canal or disc. It is the smaller of the two openings that can be made in the lamina. (Refer to Illustration 9.1 on the following page.)

<u>Laminectomy</u> (lamb-in-eck-toe-me) means to *completely* remove the thin bony plate. For example, if a vertebral disc has herniated, the surgeon may need to remove pieces of the fragmented disc. When the vertebra's lamina is out of the way, greater access to the disc is facilitated. (Refer to Illustration 9.2 on page 126.)

Either one of these two surgical procedures enlarges the natural window, thereby providing greater access to the spinal canal or other related anatomical parts. The offending element (i.e. osteophytes, disc debris, etc.) can be seen more easily and removed.

◆ ◆ ◆ ◆ ◆

ILLUSTRATION 9.1

LAMINOTOMY

-Posterior View of Spine-

A laminotomy removes just a portion of the lamina. The procedure enables the surgeon to have greater access to the underlying canal, disc, and/or nerves.

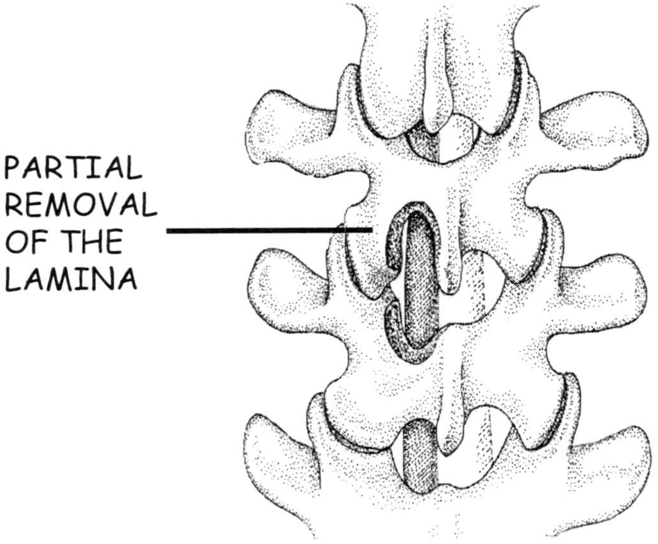

ILLUSTRATION 9.2

LAMINECTOMY

-Posterior View of Spine-

A laminectomy removes the entire lamina. If spinal stenosis is present, the surgeon may enlarge the 'window', or neuroforamen, to allow room for nerves to exit.

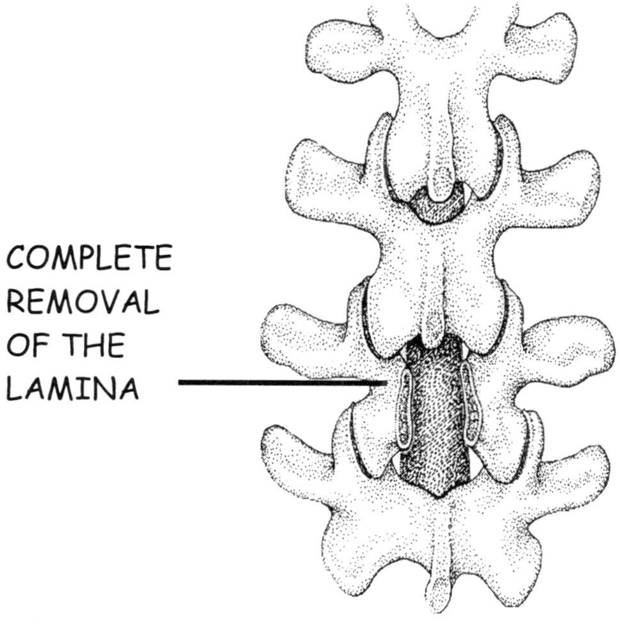

FORAMINOTOMY

A *foraminotomy* (for-aye-men-ott-toe-me) is a particular type of surgical procedure that may be used to treat foraminal spinal stenosis. If the foramen (for-aye-men, *window*) becomes clogged with debris, nerve roots may become irritated resulting in inflammation.

The surgeon uses small tools to *shave* open the inside of the foramen increasing its size. Once the nerves have ample space, and compression has been eliminated, the inflammation and associated pain may diminish. The *open* windows allow the nerves exiting the spinal column to easily slip through the foramen.

◆ ◆ ◆ ◆ ◆

SPINAL INSTRUMENTATION and FUSION

Spinal instrumentation is a generic term for surgical procedures that incorporate the use of screws, rods, cages, plates, and/or cylinders. These pieces are termed *hardware*. (Refer to Illustration 9.3 on page 130.)

Fusion simply means the addition of bone (bone graft) and may be used in conjunction with hardware. When fusion and hardware are combined, it can provide structural support where the spine has failed. Fusion is similar concrete (bone grafts) reinforced with steel (instrumentation).

When redundant vertebral motion (same repeated action) places constant pressure on surrounding nerves, pain may result. Fusion stops the movement and either eliminates or reduces the pain.

With spinal instrumentation and fusion working together, the patient may be able to get up the day following surgery. Before hardware was available, bone grafting (bone tissue) simply was not enough to provide immediate spinal stability. In those days, the patient was put into a plaster body cast to hold everything still so the area could fuse. Using hardware, the bone actually may grow around the rods and/or other hardware ... similar to reinforced concrete.

Fortunately patients are no longer placed in plaster casts following back surgery. Sometimes the physician will order a corset or non-rigid support designed to limit spinal motion. These brace-like supports are intended to restrict movement much like a splint. They are worn on a short-term basis. As soon as an x-ray proves fusion has occurred, the use of the brace may be discontinued.

In a severe case of degenerative disc disease, a vertebral disc may be removed. Once the disc is gone, a space remains between the two vertebral bodies creating an unstable spine. A ***cage*** (similar to a tiny birdcage) may be filled with bone tissue and inserted into the empty disc space. Bone graft is packed around the cage within the once empty space. (Refer to Illustration 9.4 on page 131.)

If a cage is not used, rods and screws are utilized and the bone tissue is laid across the hardware. In either case, the vertebrae are assisted in growing together to form a solid block of bone.

Some people think that their spine will be stiff as a board after fusion. However, this is not true. Consider the mechanics of standing up and sitting down. Most of the motion occurs in the hip joints, not in the spine.

Fusion will not prohibit the patient from bending over, but it will limit a portion of the spine's motion. The trade-off is acceptable because after fusion pain from movement may be eliminated or reduced.

For patients who are at high risk for failed fusion (such as smokers), bone growth stimulators may be used. Stimulators are either placed internally complete with a battery (similar to a pacemaker) or worn externally like a belt.

These devices emit electromagnetic waves, which may promote the healing of bone tissue. However, just because these devices are available does not mean that all high-risk patients are suited for fusion.

◆ ◆ ◆ ◆ ◆

ILLUSTRATION 9.3

SPINAL INSTRUMENTATION and FUSION

Hardware (rods, screws, etc.) is combined to stabilize the spine.

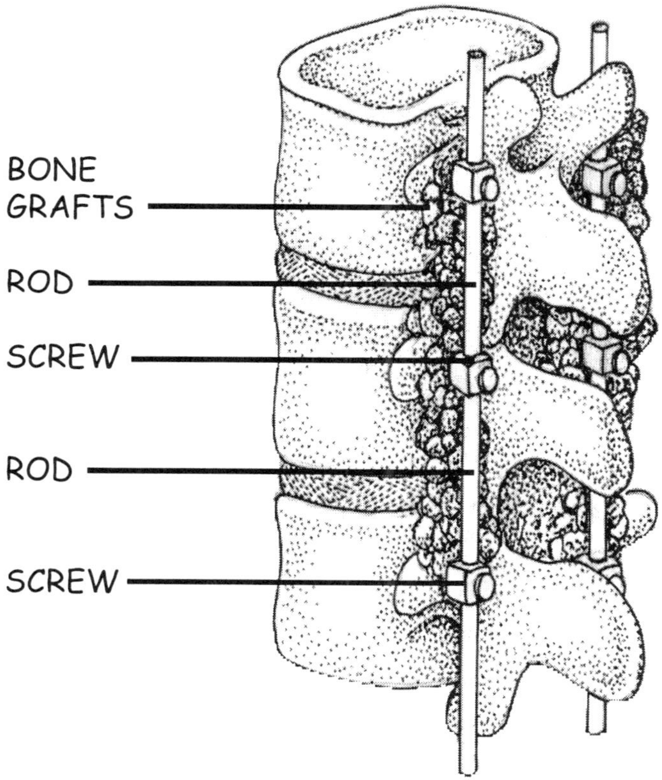

ILLUSTRATION 9.4

THE 'CAGE'

The cage is used to fill and stabilize the disc space created by disease and/ or the removal of a vertebral disc. A cage can be made from bony material or a metal alloy.

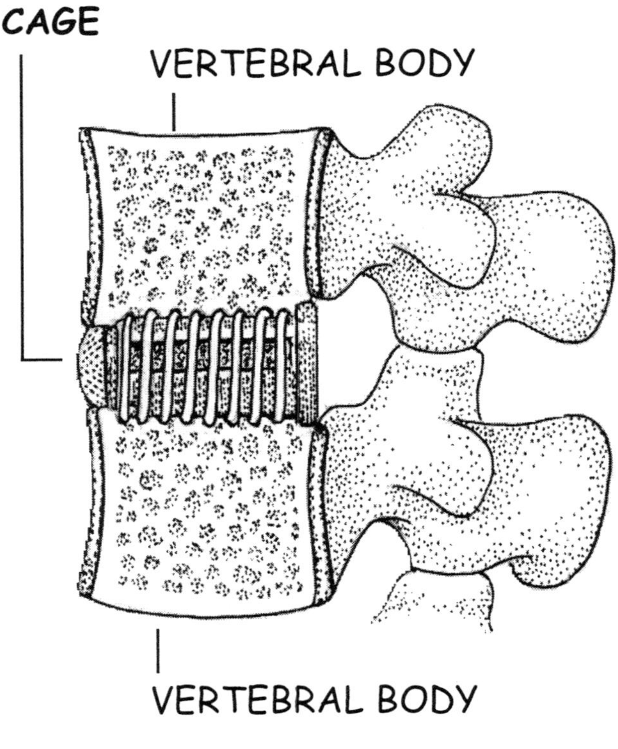

THE FUTURE OF SPINAL SURGERY

A Trend Toward Less Invasive Procedures

The trend in spinal surgery is moving toward less invasive procedures. A similar trend started with knee surgery some 20 years ago. At that time, if a patient had torn knee cartilage the surgical procedure required opening the knee. It took several weeks, if not months, for the patient to recover.

Now many knee surgeries are performed through an *arthroscopic* tube (are-throw-sca-pick) enabling the patient to rapidly recover. Medical technology continues to develop smaller surgical instruments allowing for smaller incisions.

Similar advances are being made in spinal surgery. Devices are now available that utilize microscopic fiber optics. The apparatus is similar to a mini TV camera capable of transmitting images to a monitor-like screen. This specialized equipment has built-in magnification, which enables the surgeon to view tiny structures inside the spine through a small hole.

THE 'CAGE'

Although artificial disc replacement has not become available, the cage (discussed on page 128) is now being used to fill disc space after a disc has been removed. (Refer to Illustration 9.4 on page 131.)

The cage is made of either a bone material or alloy metals. It may be filled with bone graft and placed into the space once occupied by a vertebral disc. Additional bone graft may be packed around the cage to provide spinal stability once healed.

◆ ◆ ◆ ◆ ◆

ARTIFICIAL DISC REPLACEMENT ... ALMOST

There has been considerable research on artificial disc replacement. At this time, artificial discs are undergoing clinical trials in various parts of the world. Emphasis has been placed on finding biological solutions for many spinal problems, especially in the area of artificial discs or disc-like substances.

It is suspected that within the next few years spinal surgeons will have an artificial disc available that is just as reliable as an artificial knee or hip. Although this is only in the experimental phase, it remains exciting news for patients who may require disc replacement in the future.

It would certainly be another milestone for medical science and technology to provide an artificial means of replacing defective body components.

◆ ◆ ◆ ◆ ◆

SOLVING THE PROBLEM OF SCAR TISSUE

Scar tissue has always been a possible problem after surgery. In some cases following a spinal procedure, the surrounding nerves may become ensnared by scar tissue.

The traditional approach to this problem was to transplant fatty tissue around the nerve root. Now technology has come to the rescue with new substances that can be applied around the nerve root to decrease the chance of scarring. These substances are now being tried and vigorously implemented in surgical procedures in North America.

◆ ◆ ◆ ◆ ◆

DIAGNOSTICALLY SPEAKING ...

The value of MRI imaging studies continues to grow. Technological advancements in computerization have made the MRI scanner faster and more compatible with patient needs. Open scanners are particularly patient-friendly to individuals who are claustrophobic.

continued ...

Technology has more recently developed a technique that produces full color three-dimensional (3-D) images of the body's anatomy. Combined with highly specialized computer software, images can be rotated and moved giving the physician heightened insight into a patient's disorder. This new tool is proving quite valuable in rendering models used in reconstructive surgeries.

◆ ◆ ◆ ◆ ◆

IN SUMMARY ...

It could be said that the practice of orthopaedics has advanced light years from the period of 1895, when Wilhelm Roentgen discovered the x-ray. Patients and physicians alike have more to look forward to than the mind can imagine.

◆ ◆ ◆ ◆ ◆

The Authors' Last Words ...

The development of new treatment options for disorders affecting the spine has certainly hit the fast track. The Palm Beach Orthopaedic and Spinal Research Foundation will continue to keep pace with these technological advancements to treat spinal disorders.

We invite each reader to share his or her comments about this book. If we have not answered your question(s), we would like to know so these issues can be addressed in future editions.

◆ ◆ ◆ ◆ ◆

Chapter 10

Glossary of Terms

ACUPUNCTURE (acc-you-punk-chur)
A practitioner inserts needles into the body at specific points to restore inner harmony and control pain.

ADRENAL HORMONE (a-dree-nal)
Estrogen, an adrenal hormone, is produced by the adrenal gland and is necessary for healthy bones.

ANALGESIC (an-all-gee-sick)
A medication used for pain control.

ANESTHESIOLOGIST (ann-es-thee-zee-all-oh-gist)
A doctor who administers sedatives and pain medication during surgical procedures.

ANKYLOSIS (an-key-low-sis)
A disease causing the spine to lose flexibility and stiffen.

ANTERIOR LONGITUDINAL LIGAMENT
A spinal ligament that attaches to the front of each vertebra.

ANTI-DEPRESSANT A prescription drug used to alleviate depression and anxiety.

ANTI-INFLAMMATORY
A drug that reduces swelling/inflammation.

ANULUS (ann-you-luss)
The tough tire-like outer layer of a vertebral disc.

ARACHNOID (ar-ack-noyd) One of the protective membranes covering the spinal cord.

ARTHRITIS (arth-rye-tis)
A common joint disease causing inflammation and pain.

BIOFEEDBACK An alternative therapy based on the theory that the patient is able to control his or her pain to a degree.

BONE GRAFTS/GRAFTING
Harvested bone used in spinal fusion procedures.

BONE SCAN A diagnostic imaging tool.

BONE STIMULATOR
A device designed to stimulate bones to heal/grow.

BONY OVERGROWTH or BONE SPUR
An abnormal bony growth resulting from disease.

BRACE A custom-fitted removable support worn to stabilize the spine.

BULGING DISC Occurs when the anulus of a vertebral disc protrudes with the nucleus pulposus intact. Also known as a Contained Disc.

CAGE
A specific type of hardware used to fill empty disc space.

CALCIFICATION (kals-eye-fi-cay-shun)
A body process that causes bone to harden.

CALLUS A granular material the body makes and deposits at the site of a fracture to help mend a fracture.

CANCELLOUS (cancel-luss) The interior compartment of bone resembling latticework.

CANNULA (can-you-la) Surgical instruments are passed through this small metal tube during percutaneous and laser procedures.

CARTILAGE (car-till-edge)
A smooth coating covering (bonded to) joint surfaces.

CAUDA EQUINA (caw-dah e-queen-ah) Part of the spinal cord resembing a horse's tail, which begins near the first lumbar vertebra.

CEREBROSPINAL FLUID (sir-ee-bro-spinal)
The liquid cushion within the layers of the spinal cord.

CERVICAL SPINE (sir-vick-all)
The first seven vertebrae starting at the base of the skull.

CHIROPRACTIC (kie-row-pra-tick) A therapy based on the body's ability to heal itself through manual manipulation of the vertebrae.

CHRONIC Mild to severe continuous pain .

CLAUSTROPHOBIC (claw-stro-foe-bick)
Fear of being in a closed place.

CLINICAL SYMPTOMS
Symptoms that define a particular disease.

COCCYX (cock-six) The last bone formation below the sacrum; also known as the tailbone.

COLLAGEN (coll-ah-gin) A protein manufactured by the body used to mend a fracture.

COMPRESSION FRACTURE
A fracture that may cause a vertebra to collapse.

COMPRESSIVE NEUROPATHY (ner-awe-path-ee)
Pressure on nerves that may cause swelling and pain.

COMPUTERIZED AXIAL TOMOGRAPHY
(CT SCAN or CAT SCAN) (tom-og-graf-ee)
A diagnostic imaging tool that uses multiple x-ray beams to produce slice-type images.

CONGENITAL Present at birth (such as a disorder).

CONTAINED DISC See Bulging Disc.

CORTICAL (core-tea-cul)
The outer layer of bone resembling concentric rings.

DEGENERATIVE DISC DISEASE A biochemical change associated with aging that may cause discs to lose moisture, crack, and/or become thin.

DERMATOMES (dur-ma-tomes)
The nerve system that supplies sensation to skin.

DIAGNOSIS The name of the disorder.

DISC A cushion-like shock absorber located between two vertebrae.

DISCECTOMY (dis-eck-toe-me) Surgical removal of a portion of or an entire intervertebral disc.

DISCOGRAPHY (diss-ah-graw-fee) A specific type of x-ray revealing the pathology of discs.

DURA MATER (dur-ah matter)
One of the outer protective layers of the spinal cord.

ELECTRICAL STIMULATION A modality that forces a muscle or muscle group to contract and relax. Stimulates circulation, may alleviate swelling, pain, and enhance healing.

ELECTROMYOGRAPHY (EMG)
(elec-tro-my-ah-graw-fee) A test used to determine normal (or abnormal) muscle function.

EPIDURAL (ep-eye-dur-all) A type of nerve block injected into and around the spinal canal or epidural space in the spine.

FACET JOINT (fah-set) The joints in the spine that enable the body to bend and twist.

FLUOROSCOPIC GUIDANCE (floor-oh-ska-pic) An imaging tool allowing a surgical procedure to be seen as it is performed.

FORAMINAL STENOSIS (for-aye-men-al sten-oh-sis) A narrowing or closing of a spinal foramen.

FORAMINOTOMY (for-aye-men-ott-toe-me) A surgical procedure performed to increase the size of the foramen.

FRACTURE Broken bone.

GENERAL ANESTHESTICS (ann-es-tha-ticks) Drugs used by an anesthesiologist during surgery that temporarily disable nerve impulses making the patient unconscious and pain free.

HARDWARE Rods, screws, and plates used in spinal instrumentation procedures.

HERNIATED DISC (her-knee-ate-it) The anulus breaks open and the nucleus pulposus leaks out. A Non-Contained Disc.

HYDROTHERAPY
Water therapy similar to a whirlpool.

HYPERFLEXION (hi-per-flex-shun) Spinal movement beyond normal (forward, backward, sideways).

IDIOPATHIC SCOLIOSIS
(id-dee-oh-path-ick sko-lee-oh-sis)
The childhood version of scoliosis.

INFLAMMATION (in-fla-may-shun) Swelling.

INFORMED CONSENT A document the patient signs after full disclosure of a medical procedure.

KYPHOSIS (ki-foe-sis) A disease that, when excessive, may cause a hump to form in the shoulder blade area of the upper back.

LAMINA (lamb-in-ah)
The thin bony plate that protects the spinal canal.

LAMINECTOMY (lamb-in-eck-toe-me)
The surgical removal of the lamina.

LAMINOTOMY (lamb-in-ah-toe-me)
The surgical removal of a portion of the lamina.

LASER (lay-zer) A surgical tool that uses an infrared source to divide or destroy tissue.

LIGAMENT Fibrous strong tissue connecting to bone, cartilage, and other structures to support the spine.

LIGAMENTUM FLAVUM (lee-ga-men-tum flay-vum) A ligament structure forming a protective hood over the dura mater connecting under the facet joints.

LOCAL ANESTHETICS (ann-es-tha-ticks) An injection at or near the procedure site to block the pain impulses sent to the brain.

LORDOSIS (lor-doe-sis) A spinal disorder that may cause the low back to curve excessively inward. Also known as swayback.

LUMBAR SPINE (lum-bar) The five vertebrae that start after the last thoracic vertebra.

MAGNET THERAPY Used to enhance circulation, promote healing, and alleviate pain. The magnets are laid on the effected area.

MAGNETIC RESONANCE IMAGING (MRI) A diagnostic imaging tool that produces detailed images without radiation.

MARROW The semi-soft center of bone responsible for the production of red blood cells.

METASTASIZE (ma-tax-ta-size) Spread to another area (such as cancer).

MICRODISCECTOMY (micro-dis-eck-toe-me) Surgical removal of a portion of or an entire vertebral disc using microscopic magnification.

MODALITY (mow-dal-it-tee) A treatment or therapy that does not require patient participation.

MUSCLE SPASM
Involuntary muscle movement due to trauma.

MYOFASCIAL RELEASE (my-oh-face-shall)
Localized massage to manipulate the fascia.

NARCOTIC
A prescription drug designed to control pain.

NERVE BLOCK INJECTION Medication is injected around nerves to decrease inflammation and pain.

NERVE CONDUCTION STUDY (NCS)
A sensitive test used to determine a nerve's ability to transmit an impulse.

NEUROFORAMEN (nur-row for-aye-men)
Window-like openings that allow nerves to exit the spine.

NEUTRAL SPINE The natural curve of the spine.

NON-CONTAINED DISC See Herniated Disc.

NUCLEUS PULPOSUS (new-clee-us pull-po-sus)
The gel-like center of a vertebral disc.

OSTEOARTHRITIS (os-tea-oh-arth-rye-tis)
The degenerative form of arthritis.

OSTEOPHYTES (os-tea-oh-fights)
Extra bone the body produces to stop joint movement.

OSTEOPOROSIS (os-tea-oh-pour-oh-sis)
A disease that causes bones to lose density.

OUTPATIENT SURGERY Same day surgery.

PALPATION (pal-pay-shun) The hands and fingers are used to place pressure on certain areas of skin to feel for what lies underneath. Skin temperature and color is also noted.

PARS ARTICULARIS (par-z are-tick-you-layer-es)
Part of the posterior vertebra, including the facet joints, that attach to the vertebral body.

PATIENT CONTROLLED ANALGESIA (PCA)
A pumping device used by some post-operative patients to alleviate pain.

PERCUTANEOUS SURGERY (per-cue-tain-ee-us)
A surgical procedure performed through a small hole made in the patient's skin.

PERIPHERAL NEUROPATHY
(per-if-fur-all ner-awe-path-ee)
A degenerative disease effecting the nerves branching into the extremities.

PHYSICAL THERAPY A conservative treatment program designed to meet a patient's functional goals.

POSTERIOR The rear. (i.e. rear view of the spine).

POSTERIOR LONGITUDINAL LIGAMENT
A ligament that runs downward, vertically, behind, and inside the spinal canal.

RADIATE (ray-dee-ate) Pain or sensation that travels away from the point of origin.

RADIOGRAPH Another term for an X-Ray.

RECOVERY ROOM A medically supervised area where a patient is moved following surgery.

REFLEXOLOGY (reflex-all-low-gee)
Similar to acupuncture except the practitioner uses the fingers and thumbs to apply pressure to specific points on the body to promote natural healing.

RHEUMATOID ARTHRITIS (RA)
(room-ah-toyed arth-rye-tis)
Progressive arthritis that can be painfully destructive.

ROOTLETS (root-lets)
Nerve roots that shoot off from the spinal cord.

RUPTURED DISC
Medically known as a herniated disc.

SACRUM (say-crumb) Triangular shaped bone mass located below the last lumbar vertebra.

SCIATICA (sy-attic-ka)
A compressive neuropathy involving the sciatic nerve.

SCOLIOSIS (sko-lee-oh-sis)
A disease that may cause the spine to curve to the side, usually into the shape of an 'S' or a 'C'.

SEDATIVE
A drug to relax and/or make the patient drowsy.

SENSORY Physical feeling.

SLIPPED DISC A layperson's term for a ruptured disc, but medically known as a herniated or bulging disc.

SOFT TISSUE INJURY
Injury to non-bony and/or non-disc portions of the spine.

SPINAL FUSION/
SPINAL INSTRUMENTATION
A surgical procedure using hardware (instrumentation) and bone grafts (fusion) to stabilize the spine.

SPINAL MENINGITIS (men-in-gi-tis)
An infection causing inflammation of the membranes in the brain and/or spinal cord.

SPINAL STENOSIS (sten-oh-sis)
A narrowing or closing of the neuroforamen (window(s)) that may cause nerve compression and pain.

SPINAL TUMOR
A rare disorder than can cause intense pain.

SPONDYLOLISTHESIS (spon-dill-oh-liss-thee-sis)
A disorder that results when one vertebra slips over another.

SPRAIN/STRAIN Occurs when a muscle, ligament, or tendon is stretched beyond its normal limits.

SUBLUXATION (sub-lux-aye-shun)
A chiropractic term meaning a spinal joint is misaligned.

SYNOVIAL FLUID (sin-no-vee-all)
A fluid that lubricates joints and nourishes cartilage.

TAILBONE Same as the Coccyx.

TENDON
A sturdy band of tissue that attaches muscle to bone.

THORACIC SPINE (thor-a-sick)
The 12 vertebrae following the last cervical vertebra.

TRIGGER POINT INJECTION
An injection at the site of pain.

ULTRASOUND A modality used to relax tight muscles, promote deep warmth, circulation, and healing.

VERTEBRA (ver-tea-bra) (singular)
VERTEBRAE (ver-tea-bray) (plural)
VERTEBRAL (ver-tea-brawl) (relating to a vertebra)
One (or more) of the 33 bones in the spinal column.

WHIPLASH
An intensive soft tissue injury to the neck.

X-RAY
A common diagnostic imaging tool using radiation to create a picture of a body part.

◆ ◆ ◆ ◆ ◆

INDEX

Acupuncture, 108, 110, 137
Acute pain, 88, 120
Alternative therapies, 108-110
Analgesic, 111, 137
Anesthetics, 118, 142, 144
Ankylosis, 76, 137
Anti-depressant, 90, 138
Anti-inflammatory, 88, 89, 111, 138
Anulus, 12, 17, 67-70, 138
Aquatic exercise, 99
Arthritis, 41, 59, 71-72, 74, 76, 97, 138
Arthroscopic, 132
Artificial disc replacement, 132-133
Bilateral response, 33
Biofeedback, 109, 138
Body mechanics, 46, 101-107
Bone density scan, 42, 84
Bone graft, 61, 127, 128, 130, 133, 138
Bone growth stimulator, 129, 138
Bone scan, 41, 138
Bony overgrowth, bone spur, 51, 72, 73-74, 81, 138
Brace, 58, 128, 138
Bulging disc, 50, 67, 70, 139 (also see Contained disc)
Cage, 128-133, 139
Calcification, 7, 58, 139
Callus, 58, 139
Cancellous, 8, 139
Cannula, 122, 139
Cartilage, 16, 23, 74, 132, 139
Cauda equina, 17, 18, 20-21, 139

Cerebrospinal fluid, 18-19, 139
Cervical, 9, 11-14, 49, 77, 139
Chiropractic, 109, 140
Chronic pain, 83, 88, 120, 140
Coccyx, 9-11, 13-14, 140
Collagen, 7, 58, 140
Compressive neuropathy, 50-51, 140
Computed axial tomography (CT or CAT scan), 38-39, 140
Congenital, 58, 61, 76, 140
Contained disc, 67, 140 (also see Bulging disc)
Cortical, 8, 141
Deep tendon reflexes, 33
Degenerative disc disease, 3, 80-81, 113, 141
Dermatomes, 18-19, 22, 141
Diagnosis, 27, 33, 88-89, 141
Diagnostic tests, 31, 34-44
Disc, 12, 39, 51, 67, 74, 80-82, 122, 132-133, 141
Discectomy, 123, 141
Discography, 43, 141
Dura mater, 16, 141
Electrical stimulation, 95-97, 141
Electromyography (EMG), 43, 141
Epidural, 53, 90, 142
Exercise, 86, 95, 98-101
Facet (joints), 16, 55, 57, 72, 74, 142
Fascia, 98
Ferromagnetic, 41
Fluoroscopic guidance, 122, 142
Foramen, 79, 80, 127 (also see Neuroforamen)
Foraminal stenosis, 50, 79, 142
Foraminotomy, 59, 79, 127, 142

Fracture, 55-58, 83-84, 140, 142
Fusion, 61, 127-130, 148
Hardware, 61, 127-130, 142
Heat treatment, 97-98
Herniated disc, 50, 67-69, 122-124, 142
(also see Non-contained disc)
Hydrotherapy, 99, 143
Hyperextension, 49
Hyperflexion, 57, 143
Ice treatment, 99
Idiopathic scoliosis, 62-63, 143
Infection, 41, 53-54
Informed consent, 116, 143
Kyphosis, 62, 65, 143
Laboratory tests, 44
Lamina, 124-126, 143
Laminectomy, 61, 124, 126, 143
Laminotomy, 51, 124-125, 143
Laser, 122, 143
Ligament, 23-24, 28, 47-49, 143
Lordosis, 62, 66, 144
Lumbar, 9-14, 77, 144
Magnetic resonance imaging (MRI), 39-41, 134, 144
Magnets, 109, 144
Medical history, 32, 35, 86, 94, 116-117
Meningitis, 54, 148
Microdiscectomy, 123, 144
Minimally invasive, 90, 116, 121-122
Modality, 96, 98, 145
Muscle, 2, 5, 24-26, 28, 33, 47-49, 83, 95, 97, 101
Muscle spasm, 48, 54, 96-97, 145
Myofascial release, 95, 98, 145

Narcotic, 89, 145
Nerve block injection, 90, 111, 145
Nerve conduction study (NCS), 43, 145
Nerve root, 9-10, 17-21, 28, 57, 69-70, 72-73, 77-79, 81, 147
Neuroforamen, 15, 18, 23, 59, 72, 76-77, 79-80, 82, 126-127, 145
Nicotine, 4, 113-114 (also see Smoking)
Non-contained disc, 67, 145 (also see Herniated disc)
Nucleus pulposus, 12, 17, 67-70, 145
Osteoarthritis, 74-75, 99, 113, 145
Osteophytes, 72, 74, 81, 124, 146
Osteoporosis, 5, 42, 57, 82-85, 146
Pain diagram, 29-31
Pain management, 87-91
Palpation, 34, 146
Patient controlled analgesia (PCA), 91, 146
Percutaneous, 121-122, 146
Peripheral neuropathy, 51, 146
Physical examination, 31, 33
Physical therapy, 5, 48, 61, 91-107, 111, 116, 120, 146
Posture, 101-107 (also see Body mechanics)
Radiate, 32, 50, 53-54, 147
Radiograph, 38, 147
Range of motion, 95, 98, 100
Reflexology, 110, 147
Rheumatoid arthritis (RA), 76, 147
Ruptured disc, 67, 123, 147
Sacrum, 9-11, 13-14, 21, 147
Scar tissue, 48, 98, 134
Sciatica, 34-35, 42, 50-52, 59, 148
Scoliosis, 2, 61-64, 95, 148
Slipped disc, 50, 67, 148

Smoking, 4-5, 83-84, 113, 129 (also see Nicotine)
Spinal canal, 16, 18, 23, 43, 50, 59, 68, 124
Spinal cord, 16, 19-20, 55, 57, 78
Spinal stenosis, 59, 76-79, 113, 126, 148
Spinal tumor, 41, 86, 149
Spinal instrumentation, 61, 127-128, 130, 148
Spondylolisthesis, 58-59, 60-61, 149
Spontaneous fracture, 83-84
Sprain, strain, 46-47, 149
Stenosis, 3, 50
Synovial fluid, 16, 149
Tailbone, 10, 149
Tendon, 24, 28, 47-49, 149
Thoracic, 9, 11-14, 149
Trigger point injection, 90, 149
Ultrasound, 95-96, 149
Vertebra, vertebrae, vertebra, 9, 11, 13, 15, 17, 55-60, 75, 82-83, 85, 128, 130-131, 133, 150
Whiplash, 49, 150
X-Ray, 37-38, 58, 63, 150

SAVE YOUR ACHING BACK

A Patient's Guide

Ordering Information

Books may be ordered directly from the publisher through its Internet website or, by mail at the address below. If you or your organization is interested in purchasing copies for promotional or educational use, volume discounts are available for bulk orders.

Single copies @ $14.95 US or $19.95 CAN each. Please include the appropriate amount for shipping and handling:

Standard (2 to 6 business days)	$3.95
Priority Mail (2 to 3 days)	$5.95

email: www.syapress.com

SYA Press, Inc.

1355 West Palmetto Park Road, Suite 115

Boca Raton, FL 33486

Please direct your comments or questions to the website or in writing to the address above.